THE NEW WAY TO RELAX

Here is a practical handbook which teaches you scores of commonsense techniques for releasing tension and getting the most out of your energy and out of your life. Follow these simple, tested methods that have helped thousands and you can feel better, look better, and enjoy life far more than you do now.

Karin Roon, an expert in applied relaxation, explains step by step how to analyse your daily habits and your surroundings and get at the causes of your tension. Insomnia, chronic fatigue, headaches, eyestrain, pains in the neck, shoulders, back, legs, arms and other parts of the body—these and similar troubles rooted in nervous and muscular tension are traced to their sources, and you are told what you can do to relieve and even eliminate them. Easy techniques of self-massage are also given. No expensive gadgets or hours or drill are required—all you need are just a few minutes a day. Clear, entertaining diagrams show exactly how to obtain relief.

This is not a book of theories—it is simple, down-to-earth commonsense.

The
New Way to Relax

by Karin Roon

With an Introduction by
Arthur Langstadt, M.D.

Illustrated by
Jesse Jacobs

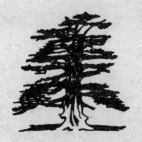

CEDAR BOOKS
An imprint of William Heinemann Limited

Published by Cedar Books
an imprint of
William Heinemann Limited
10 Upper Grosvenor Street, London W1X 9PA
LONDON   MELBOURNE   TORONTO
JOHANNESBURG   AUCKLAND
Copyright © Karin Roon
All rights reserved
First published 1951
First published as a Cedar Book 1956
This impression 1986

0 434 11114 7

Printed in Great Britain by
Richard Clay (The Chaucer Press) Ltd,
Bungay, Suffolk

Introduction

THE medical profession has come increasingly to recognise tension as an underlying cause in many illnesses. Our neurotic age is in urgent need of practical help for the many people who are over-stimulated and fear-ridden.

This book by Karin Roon provides such practical help. It is easy to understand and it can be applied by anyone who really wants to help himself. The author's wide experience and the human feeling that brightens every chapter make the book fascinating reading. Mrs. Roon's new approach to the correction of bad habits is interesting, and if her suggestions are carefully followed, functional damage can be forestalled.

I am glad to see a discussion of breathing habits—hitherto neglected—brought into the foreground, as I have watched the beneficial results on my own patients after childbirth from practising correct breathing, particularly in its effect on the restoration of correct posture and muscle flexibility.

ARTHUR LANGSTADT, M.D.

CONTENTS

vii

About This Book

THIS book has been written in order to reach a larger audience than I can meet through personal treatments, or in classes, or over the radio, or on the lecture platform. After many years of experience, I have come to the conclusion that millions of people are defrauding themselves of the health, energy, happiness, and development of their own powers that they might achieve simply by learning how to get the most out of their own bodies. It is too often worry and tension and unhappiness that make us suffer, not illness that wreaks this havoc upon us.

Although the purpose of this book is to show you that you can accomplish more by taking it easy, there are certain categories of people who should not attempt to follow it without the supervision of their physicians: these are people who suffer from serious heart conditions or from high and low blood-pressure. Nor should the work be undertaken by anyone with tuberculosis.

I suggest that you first read the book through from beginning to end. Then go back to the beginning and take it up chapter by chapter, conscientiously trying each suggestion for yourself. You may have to try several times before you can do each of these new techniques properly, but when you master them you will feel for yourself that they relieve tension, rest you, and improve your spirits and attitude of mind.

If you are suffering from serious tension, your condition is the result of months, or perhaps even many years, of wrong functional habits, wrong ways of living. In that case, it would be unreasonable to expect to feel "as good as new" within a few days or even a few weeks. You will discover, however, that you experience almost immediate temporary relief. What

I want this book to do for you—what it can do if you are willing to observe your own habits carefully for a comparatively short time—is to bring about a lasting relief from tension, a new awareness of yourself as a person, and an ability to live through twenty-four hours every day with a new capacity for enjoyment, with new courage, and with a deep conviction that your life makes sense and that it is worth living.

KARIN ROON

CHAPTER ONE

You Can Relax!

WHY should there be a guide for adults, dealing with the problems of tension and relaxation? Because tension is everybody's complaint. People feel that something is wrong with them, they complain of pain and fatigue, they are depressed and irritable, they dread life instead of enjoying it, they evade it instead of facing it.

It is for these people that this book has been written, for the thousands who go to over-worked doctors or over-crowded hospitals for help and are told: "There is nothing wrong with you. Just take it easy and relax."

Is there nothing wrong with you? Well, there is nothing that medical science can detect in tests and examinations. What is wrong is the functioning of your body in everyday life, the kind of use and abuse you give it, the wear and tear of certain muscle groups, the neglect of certain others. Little things.

If your body were an automobile you would not be permitted to drive it—for your own safety and that of your fellow men—until you learned how to handle it properly. Unless you are an exceptionally fortunate person, however, you have never been taught how to use your body to the best advantage: how, in the language of the automobile, to get the most mileage out of your petrol; how to avoid over-taxing your motor; how to get a smooth-running performance without a lot of rattles.

People often feel that they are helpless—and hopeless—victims of inferior bodies. If they had only been born with more energy or straighter backs, with firmer muscles or better nerves, everything would be fine. But if you look around, you will observe that it is not always the finest car that goes

I

farthest and with the least trouble; it is the car with the best driver.

The over-burdened doctor who checks your heart and your lungs and your blood-pressure has little time to devote to the functioning of your body. Certainly, he is unlikely to ask you any of the following questions:

1. Do you wake up tired and listless in the morning?
2. Are you afraid of what the day may hold for you?
3. Do you feel irritable?
4. Do you suffer from stiff shoulders and a tired back, from nagging aches and pains?
5. Do you feel rushed, as though you were always a little behind?
6. Are you over-burdened, knowing that you have undertaken more than you can handle?
7. Do you suffer from a sense of fatigue and exhaustion that leaves you depressed?
8. Are you dragged down by a sense of personal failure and discouragement?
9. Are you a chronic worrier?
10. Do you know how to use your body and how to plan your life?

Scientists have discovered that tension is the underlying cause in many physical and mental diseases. Out of my own studies and experience has grown a conviction that tension, because of its effect on the organs of the body and general health, is the great killer after middle age; that it is at the root of much of our child delinquency, and the cause of many personality distortions, frustrations, and widespread unhappiness.

The purposes of this book are:

1. To show you why you become tense, what effect tension has on your body, how you can eliminate tension and avoid it in the future.

2. To help you analyse your daily life habits and show you that they are a clue to relaxation or tension, to proper or improper body function.

3. To teach you to correct your bad habits and provide you with techniques for self-massage, for the proper development of under-worked muscle groups, and the release of over-worked muscles.

4. To teach you to understand the car you drive through life, so that you can handle it correctly, improve your general health, overcome insomnia, and prevent future illnesses.

5. To show you, step by step, how to live on twenty-four hours a day so that you will get the most out of your energy and the most out of your life.

6. To show you how to get more satisfaction out of your sex life.

7. To point out the techniques by which the middle-aged can acquire new vitality and a sense of rejuvenation; get rid of double chins and flabby tissue.

8. To show you how to develop the full potentialities of your personality.

9. To show you how to win in the eternal war of nerves which a man wages with his environment.

10. To point the way to a practical method for acquiring peace of mind.

What is Tension?

But first, before we analyse the causes that create tension, let us try to find out what we mean by "being tense". The phrase frequently causes confusion because it is used to describe two different conditions: a muscular strain and a mental state.

One person may complain, "I am so tense I could scream," and mean that he is mentally afraid. Another person says, "I am tense; please relax me," and wants release of tense muscles.

The use of the same expression for two different complaints makes it necessary for us to speak of mental tension when we refer to a state of mind and of physical tension when a muscular sensation is described.

Much has been written in the last few years about mental tension; the subject of mental relaxation is uppermost in the minds of psychiatrists, psychologists, ministers and teachers. The new science of psychosomatic medicine is devoting much time and research to the problems of mental tensions. But so far, little is known about physical or muscular tension as the root not only of mental tension but of physical disease as well. And nothing at all has been said about the importance of daily living habits as the most common cause for both mental and physical tension. Little things again.

It is generally agreed that physical and mental tension are interrelated. Every mental activity affects the muscles. Every muscular tension affects the mind. Because of this fundamental relation of brain and muscles, you cannot be really healthy in mind or in body if the energies arising in the brain are either repressed or insufficiently released through your muscles.

Tension Is Unreleased Energy

The failure to release tension is caused either by faulty physical habits or by emotional maladjustment, so, in the long run, the answer to the question, "What causes tension?" is YOU.

Physically, emotionally, or mentally, you have faced problems of living which you have failed to solve, and the result is tension, which, starting with minor discomfort, with fatigue and nagging pain, can lead to almost all the diseases in the *Materia Medica.*

Sounds bad, doesn't it? But there is a bright side to the picture. The cause lies with *you,* but so does the cure. Since tension grows out of wrong habits, release of tension obviously comes from the substitution of right habits. It is the purpose of this book to analyse those wrong habits and to show you how to replace them by others that will release tension, give you increased vitality, improve your looks, and release the submerged powers in your own personality.

While our job is primarily to release muscular strain, we cannot ignore the emotional and mental factors. Every thought that passes through your mind, every emotion that you feel, affects the way in which your body behaves.

That is why an overdrawn bank account or a humiliation or the exhilaration that follows a public success can alter your heartbeat, disturb your digestion, and interfere with your breathing. The political argument that made you angry, Johnnie's mistake in cutting down the wrong tree, and the burned stew for dinner all have a physical as well as an emotional and a mental effect.

As long as our nervous energy finds an undisturbed outlet, we have no complaint. But when the normal release is blocked up, a state of tension develops and we begin to look around for help.

Tension is like a pebble thrown into a quiet pool. The ripples spread until they reach the farthest bank. They not only affect your health and your spirits, your energy and your capacity for joyous living, but they react upon your family and your friends, your co-workers and your community.

To-day, the nervous or over-tense person goes to his doctor, and there is comparatively little that his doctor can do for him. The medical profession is overwhelmed, not merely because of the increasing number of patients but because medicine has made such enormous strides in the last couple of generations that the sheer burden of acquiring all this information, or even a fraction of it, puts appalling strain upon the medical student.

If a doctor of fifty years ago could return, he would find himself in unknown country. Penicillin, sulfa drugs, vitamins, hormones, the miracles of modern surgery, would all be new to him. But in this spectacular advance, one thing has been overlooked: a knowledge of body function or use that is in harmony with modern living. The scarcity of doctors, the prodigious mass of information to be digested, the research to be

5

done on such pressing problems as cancer, have relegated the study of body function to the background.

Misused Energy

And yet, in an overwhelming proportion of cases, the root of our trouble is simply that we do not know how to use our bodies properly. We are out of harmony with our own natures. We have forgotten how to balance the outer pace at which we live with our own inborn rhythms. We have forgotten, or perhaps we have never learned, how to use our energy. Because it does not find the proper outlet, we store it up in the form of tension. The only way we know to release it is through alcohol, tobacco, or illnesses which are only symbols of mental and emotional tensions.

How often to-day we hear the expression, "I'm all mixed up". It's true. Mentally, emotionally, nervously, people are "all mixed up". But it does not occur to one person in a thousand that his mental and emotional confusion, his difficulty in concentrating, and his inability to make decisions can have a physical basis. But of course they can.

When you use unco-ordinated muscles, you create a state in your mind like that of a mixed-up switchboard. You make wrong connections and your nerve impulses get confused. If you learn how to make the muscles of your body function as they were intended to do, this crossed connection clears up and you experience a feeling of orderliness and clearness which tends to produce better concentration—the ability to follow through an idea without becoming involved in extraneous sensations or thoughts that cross the main thinking line. The person who concentrates properly can follow through and make decisions; he knows what he wants. Once you can concentrate, indeed, things seem to clear up by themselves, not only in business but in personal troubles as well.

The person who is "all mixed up" cannot make up his mind ,which means that unsolved problems accumulate, creating further tensions.

6

How long did you lie awake last night wondering what to do about the mortgage on the house or whether to tell the boss about the new idea that would revolutionise the business? Should you interfere with your daughter's plans or let her lead her own life? You couldn't make up your mind about anything. You just got more and more awake. The more you tossed the more difficult your problems looked and the more helpless you felt about facing them.

When you started out this morning, you were tense because you were aware of the problems you had failed to solve.

And what can the doctor do for you? He pats you on the head and tells you that organically you are sound. You need a change or a better diet to build you up; you need more rest or more play.

"Go home and relax," he tells you jovially.

But you don't know how to relax. You don't even know what makes you tense. And in time you go to a hospital to be treated for an illness whose basis is tension. That is the trouble with at least seventy-five per cent of the people in hospital beds to-day.

What Can You Do About It?

What, then, are you to do about the situation? It is my hope that this book will help you to find a practical answer to that question. This is not a book on "How to be your own doctor", and it is not intended to replace periodical check-ups by your physician. It is simply a working manual for every-day living.

If you expect a lot of routine, strenuous exercises, I am sorry to disappoint you. In any case, you would not carry them out long. You might start with the best intentions, but in a short time you would give up.

What I do want to teach you is the far-reaching effect of proper body function and how to relieve tension from head to toe, not as a result of long and arduous exercises, but from the first day and with the first simple, common-sense techniques.

7

When your energy begins to serve you instead of injuring you, there will be unexpected benefits in the flowering of personality, in a capacity for living fully and joyously—which is almost unknown to the majority of adults—and in a new freedom from the fears with which most of us are shackled.

For we are, as a whole, frightened people. It does no good to point out that we create our own fears, that we fight against our own peace, that we stand like shadows in the way of our own happiness, that our frustrations are of our own making and our failures often of our own deliberate choice. And yet these things are true.

We create our own sorrows, our own limitations, even our own bad health. And we can, if we will, knock off our shackles and release the misdirected energies by which we are storing up the forces of our own destruction.

What do I mean by misdirected energies? Look at the small boy who stubbornly insists on his own way; his hands are clenched, he is literally choked with rage, his muscles are tense, his face is strained. All his energy is concentrated in his bottled-up anger. Now that energy must find a natural and healthy outlet or it will explode in an unhealthy form, or he will continue to store it up in the form of tension that will result in mental or physical ill health.

If he is allowed to continue tying himself up in knots of anger, to hold his breath as many children do in a kind of threat to their parents, he will lose in time the natural ability to release tension, and in his adult years he will turn to artificial aids such as alcohol and narcotics to give him the release that he must have. He will become one of the countless thousands who drag along instead of living fully, because their energy is blocked up in tension. Or—even more trying to family and associates—this energy may be expended in the form of nervous habits.

Habits of the Tense Person

Every now and then it is a sound idea to check yourself,

8

to make a kind of inventory of the ways in which you are discharging your energy. Have you any of the following habits, which indicate that somewhere in your body or mind there is a tension that needs an outlet? *

1. Do you constantly wet your lips with the tip of your tongue?
2. Do you clamp your teeth hard together while working or reading?
3. Do you bite your nails?
4. Are you a pencil tapper?
5. Do you perform a drumbeat with your fingers on the arm of your chair.
6. Are you acquiring a nervous tic around your mouth?
7. Do you frown most of the time?
8. Do you constantly glance at your wrist-watch?
9. Do you crack your knuckles?
10. Are you a chain smoker?

In the following pages you are going to learn how to relax and how to correct your daily habits. But I must point out here that *reading a book will not relax you*. You have to do the work yourself. All that you need is a genuine desire to feel better, to get a higher rate of interest on your investment in living, and a little patience.

You did not get out of condition in a single day, it is the result of wrong function over a period of time. Learning to substitute new habits is not an overnight process, but this, at least, I can promise you: from the first day and with the first new habit you will be aware of improvement and you will feel better. Once you realise how much better you feel, nothing can stop you.

*WARNING: Do not simply try to repress the habit, which will only make you more tense. Try first to get at the cause—a muscular tension of which you were unaware, a mental irritation seeking relief in this way, or an emotional repression.

CHAPTER TWO

What Causes Tension

THE chances are that it is evening and you have settled down after dinner with this book. You may be a business man or a career girl, a housewife who has just finished the dishes and put junior to bed; you may be a college student or an elderly man or woman.

You have picked up this book because the time has come when you feel that something must be done about yourself. Perhaps there is a nagging pain in your shoulders and the back of your neck; your teeth are clamped together; you are frowning. You are aware of fatigue and irritation and a sense of frustration. At this moment, to-morrow and all the to-morrows ahead of that seem too much for you.

Part of your mind—for it is hard to concentrate when you are tense—is still on unfinished business, or a man you meant to see, or an errand you didn't have time to do. Part of your mind resents being put to work on your problem. Why not just turn on the radio, or read a mystery, or go to a movie? Why not just slip off into a pleasant dream and evade the whole situation?

But part of your mind is still on the job. Because—no fooling—you've got to get rid of your tension before it goes any farther.

Agreeable Tension

Tension is a part of normal living and, so long as it can be released, can often be an agreeable sensation. Certainly it is true that tension, of one kind or another, accompanies all the high points of our lives. There is tension in the moment of expectation before you unwrap a present, tension between two people in love before the moment of the first kiss, tension at the climax of a ball game when you fought for victory with your last reserves, tension that stimulates and carries you away at the exciting points of a play or a movie.

In other words, tension in itself is not an evil; it helps to contribute to our great moments of happiness, buoyancy and achievement.

Unreleased Tension

Tension becomes a problem only when it is unreleased. There are three sources of tension: mental, emotional, and physical. If the source is mental, the chief sensations will be those of headache, fatigue, and lack of concentration. If the source is emotional, one of the sensations may be a tightness around the ribs near the heart, a feeling of stiffness, and a more or less pronounced fear or sense of frustration. If the source is physical, the chief sensation will be pain and discomfort either in those parts of the body directly connected with the affected muscle group or in a remote part as a result of referred pain.

Mental Tension

In case the source is mental, the best remedy for the brain is rest. Often a change of surroundings, a short trip, or a new activity will break up the tension. Some people have the wonderful capacity of restoring themselves through sleep. The leading example, perhaps, is Napoleon. I recently talked with a prominent New York dentist, Dr. John B. Steinberg, who is able to take one- and two-minute naps at frequent intervals during the day, and finds them extraordinarily relaxing.

But even when you feel sure that the source of the trouble is mental over-work, you must realise that your muscles are involved. Investigation will often reveal that the real cause of your trouble is not the amount of work you are doing but the way in which you are doing it. For instance, your fatigue may be the result of bad head posture that checks the blood supply to the brain, or an obstructed nose that blocks blood circulation.

Emotional Tension

In case the source is emotional, the many branches of psychiatry and psycho-analysis try to find the deep-rooted, often subconscious, reasons for the tension, and thus help people to free themselves. Frequently, psychiatric treatment alone will bring complete relief, but in other cases the muscles involved in the tension have formed habits that fail to correct themselves even when the root of the complaint has been relieved.

Frequently, comments that psychiatric treatment has not been successful simply indicate that wrong muscular habits have become fixed and caused new tensions.

Muscular Tension

This is caused, in the physiological sense, through the inability of some muscle groups to relax. Every muscle in the human body, except the diaphragm, can perform one duty and only one duty. In order to raise your arm, you must use several muscles, while other muscles bring it down again. As long as all the muscle groups work in perfect balance, everything is well and no tension can develop.

Environmental Tension

We are all aware of the hazards of heavy traffic, of the dangers of escaping gas, of the effects on the health of such hazards as "smog", and so forth. Few of us are aware, however, of the beating which our nervous and muscular systems take, day in and day out, from much less spectacular phases of our environment.

Because of the widely varying degrees of sensitivity in people, some of us are disturbed by conditions which have no effect on others. On the whole, nearly everyone is affected to some degree by the constant impact of noise in our cities. Even sounds with which we are so familiar that we are not conscious of hearing them, affect the nervous system and cause fatigue. Recent investigations of sleep habits reveal that night noises will accelerate the heartbeat although the sleeper does not awaken.

Anyone who believes that he is so accustomed to the steady undercurrent of noise, even at night when it is never really quiet, that it does not affect him any more, discovers his error after a day or two in the country. At first, he feels uneasily that something is missing. Imperceptibly, his nerves begin to loosen up, his pace grows slower, less headlong, his voice becomes quieter.

One summer on Cape Cod I taught relaxation to a number of dramatic students, as basic training for their acting. They were all city bred, accustomed to the shrill, mechanical noises of metropolitan streets. I discovered that they actually could not hear the muted sounds of the country. Because of the constant impact of noise in their daily lives, they had learned to shut out noises in an involuntary effort to prevent constant tension.

On a quiet, sunny day I took them out to a meadow and asked them to shut their eyes and simply listen. It was interesting to watch their faces. At first they were tense and alert; then they became impatient because they heard nothing. Then, little by little, they became aware of the distant rhythm of the waves, the faint cheep of a bird, the humming of insects. And the strain fell away from their faces and the tension from their bodies while they listened to the out-of-doors and enjoyed it like music.

For the most part, we cannot avoid the noises which surround us in cities, although we can learn to cope with them.

Such noises, however, as blaring radios, should be kept under control. And I might point out here that one unrecognised source of tension is the habit of keeping a radio turned on all the time, whether or not one is deliberately listening to it. Part of the mind strains to hear even when engaged with a book or in conversation, playing havoc with concentration and stirring up confused nerve impulses. Radios should be turned on only when you are prepared to give them your full attention.

Light and Rest

Electric light may be another unrecognised source of nerve tension because of its effect on sensitive eyes. Our forebears undoubtedly suffered during the winter months from a lack of adequate light, but we to-day tend to over-expose our eyes to light.

It is interesting to observe the calming influence on nerves, mood, and voice when people eat by candlelight instead of under the glare of brilliant central lighting. Our instincts tell us to dim the lights when we want to rest, but the more civilised we grow, the less we heed our instincts and we rarely think, when we are tired after a difficult day, of turning off the brighter lights and letting a shaded lamp provide the soft glow which rests our nerves and helps us to release tension.

The Effects of Colour

Colours, too, play an unsuspected part in making our working and our home environments restful. Nearly everyone is more susceptible to colour than he realises, and investigation has shown that certain colours are stimulating while others are relaxing; that one colour may arouse dissension in people and another bring harmony. Louis Cheskin, of the Colour Research Institute of America, has discovered some fascinating effects of colour. Red, he points out, has a violently stimulating effect, while blue, the coldest of all colours, is a psychological sedative.

We are rarely conscious of the effect of colour, just as we are rarely conscious of the effect of noise. And yet it can tire us, just as the impact of noise can tire us. Louis Cheskin has related that fatigue which appeared day after day in mid-afternoon in a certain factory was eliminated by the simple process of painting the boxes on which the men worked a cheerful green instead of their original sombre black. Patients grow restless with walls of glaring white and tend to recuperate more readily when there are pastel colours around them. Some hospitals and schools are now painting their walls in soft shades with excellent results.

In time, we will learn not to decorate our rooms with a view to colour fashion or to matching a favourite piece of furniture, but with a full awareness of the fact that one colour makes us happy or brings peace, while another makes us restless and discontented.

How Comfortable Is Your Furniture?

More tangible than the effects of noise, light, and colour, are the effects of furniture on our comfort and well-being.

Our furniture, of course, is adapted to crowded living conditions, but its unfortunate effect on our health is far-reaching. Let us take the chief culprit—the studio couch which is used both as a bed and as a chair. What are its shortcomings? First, it tends to sag because it is used too much, and therefore it provides the wrong support for your back. Second, it is open at both ends, and consequently does not give you the same feeling of protection as a bed with a headboard and endpiece. Almost invariably, a person who is accustomed to sleeping on a studio couch discovers that when he sleeps in a regular bed he has a greater feeling of security.

Third, and most important, the studio couch is too small. The body of the adult, like the body of the healthy baby, should have space in which to stretch, to fling the arms and legs wide, to get all the kinks out of the muscles. When you can't swing your arm without hitting the wall or stretch your full length without falling out of bed, you are forced to abandon one of your best means of rest and relaxation.

The second offender, and a serious source of tension and bad posture habits, is the kind of chair in which too many people spend most of their waking hours. The sedentary worker spends his life sitting. Unfortunately for him, this position prevents his leg muscles and trunk and arm muscles from working and it is therefore considered the most unhealthy position of the body. And if the chair tends to throw him out of alignment, to create muscular tensions and promote fatigue, it is small wonder he begins to feel that something is wrong with him.

The White-Collar Worker

Let's do a little arithmetic together. The sedentary worker —the clerk, stenographer, business executive—starts his round of sitting at the breakfast table; spends about an hour sitting in bus, car, or Tube on his way to work, eight hours at a desk; a return trip home, and then he usually spends the evening sitting either at home, in a friend's house, or at the movies. That provides an average of sixteen hours a day in a sitting position.

The result—when posture is bad because of poor habits or a poor chair—is a lack of activity for his leg muscles and, gradually, flabby buttocks that inevitably produce a weak back, hanging shoulders and neck muscles that fail to support the head upright.

When this functional abuse continues year in and year out, it is not surprising if at length your inner organs start to complain. An inevitable result of this lack of use of so many muscles is a lack of flexibility in your trunk, muscular tension, and diminished circulation of your blood.

In the beginning there will be nothing really wrong, but you will be aware of fatigue that settles much earlier in the day than it should, a dragged-out feeling, and a loss of the zest for living. The demands of the day will seem to be too heavy to carry.

Add to these results of the sixteen-hour sitting habit the effects of a poorly designed chair and you are really in for trouble. From school to office, from theatre to home, chairs are built without adjustable heights so that the tall person and the short try to fit themselves to the chair as Procrustes fitted the travellers to his bed. The ensuing discomfort leads to bad posture habits in an effort to relieve strain, and is a chief reason for the habit of crossed legs which we will discuss later, as it in turn leads to bumps on the inside of the knees, foot trouble, lack of proper thigh development and underfunction of the lower back and buttocks. The simple things, you begin to discover, have far-reaching effects on your health and well-being.

If we've got to spend our lives sitting down, there is no sound reason why we should not have chairs made by someone who knows how a human body is built.

The Impact of People

A major cause of tension is the impact of other people upon you. This ranges from the mood of your husband or wife at the breakfast table to the irritability of your boss; from the excitability of the stranger next to you in the restaurant who made a scene which left you with indigestion, to the voices of the people in your office.

Just as a relaxed person has the ability to relax those about him, so the tense person can generate tension. The irritable employer can keep his entire organisation in a state of nerves. There are countless cases of nervous prostration due to the daily impact of tense people on others. The tense father or mother can destroy a child's emotional balance. How many psychological problems that child psychologists try to settle by

17

treating the child might be prevented if the parents themselves were to learn how to relax!

How Voices Affect Us

We are learning more and more how voices affect us. The voice that is high and shrill grates on our nerves, the voice that is angry and belligerent arouses belligerence in the listener. The flat, monotonous voice causes fatigue.

It is an interesting experiment to pay attention to your own voice and discover what its effect is on you. By altering its pitch you can frequently alter your own mood. Just as you feel and look more confident when you stand straight, so you feel and sound more confident when your voice is clear, controlled, and resonant.

1. Do you mutter in a monotone in which there is never any resonance, keeping your voice muffled so that you never hear its full, clear tone? That is a sign of frustration. Let your voice go. Don't be afraid of it.

2. Is your voice aggressive? This does not mean merely that you sound dictatorial; it may mean too that you make every statement as though that were the last word on the subject. Aggressiveness in a speaker, as I said, arouses aggressiveness in the listener.

3. Do you sound plaintive and fretful? The tone which reveals self-pity is a guaranteed non-conductor for sympathy. It is almost impossible to feel sorry for the fellow who feels sorry for himself. The worst of it is that the more plaintive you sound, the more plaintive you feel. William James made this point tellingly in his *Gospel of Relaxation:*

"The voice, for example, in a surprisingly large number of us, has a tired and plaintive sound. Some of us are really tired (for I do not mean absolutely to deny that our climate has a tiring quality); but far more of us are not tired at all, or would not be tired at all unless we had got into a wretched trick of feeling tired, by following the prevalent habits of vocalisation and expression. And if talking high and tired,

18

and living excitedly and hurriedly, would only enable us to *do* more by the way, even while breaking us down in the end, it would be different. . . ." *

The voice carries its own meanings over and above the words it speaks. Say to your small son in a loud and blustering tone, "I think you are a fine boy and I'm going to get you a bicycle," and the chances are that he will burst into tears. Snarl at your wife that she is still the only woman in the world and you will see the words carry little weight if the tone is wrong.

At a time when the spoken word is of mounting importance and reaches such vast audiences over the radio, it is important for public speakers, ministers, and teachers to familiarise themselves with the psychological effect of their voices, so that they can develop their full potentialities and vary their dynamic range.

What's Your Hurry?

And now we come to a leading cause of tension to-day. Few people have any idea of how to plan their time. Every one of us has exactly the same endowment—twenty-four hours to spend at our own discretion. It is the most important thing we have in life, but we do not learn how to balance our time budget.

Do you plan too much for one day? Do you know the average amount of time that your routine tasks should take? Do you allow a small margin for emergencies?

No one can make that time budget for you. Your requirements will vary because a man's inborn rhythm is as highly individual as his finger-prints. For some people a slow, steady pace is necessary; for others a rapid and uneven pace is best. Some have a great reserve of energy on which to draw and can work for many hours; others find that they are able to do only a small amount of work without serious fatigue.

*Included in *Talks to Teachers on Psychology: and to Students on Some of Life's Ideals*, Longmans, Green and Co. Ltd.

In the long run, that isn't really important. Charles Darwin accomplished his immense scientific work in tiny periods of time, sometimes as little as a quarter of an hour in a day; rarely more than a couple of hours, because of ill health. The essential thing is to strike your own natural pace.

The trouble with most of us is that we try to adapt our own rhythms to those of our environment. We forget that a man travels longest when he goes at his own gait. Life is not a regimented parade in which you don't dare fall out of step.

The traffic whizzes by; the man beside you rushes forward as the light changes. All right. Let him go. You don't have to keep up. When you change your pace, you change your innate rhythm and you sacrifice an important part of your own personality. In fact, *you cannot fully develop and express your own personality except in terms of your own individual rhythm.*

We drive ourselves with nervous haste. And some day in middle age we find the machinery breaking down; the rushed executive goes to the hospital with stomach ulcers, the worried business man has a heart attack, the middle-aged woman complains that she has become prematurely old, that her body is flabby and functioning poorly, that she has pain and fatigue and general discomfort, that her married life is going on the rocks.

The secret is, first, to find your own rhythm and, second, to balance your time budget to fit your rhythm. The result will be that you will release new vitality and be able to accomplish more with less effort, less haste and less fatigue. Later on, we will tell you how to do it.

Take a look at the man across from you on the bus, his face nervous and intent; at the woman who rushes past you on the pavement, frowning, breathing in quick, shallow breaths. They are in a hurry. "I haven't time to catch a breath," they exclaim if you stop them for a greeting.

And it is quite true. Frequently the thing people call nervousness is merely disturbed breathing rhythm. The breath is quick and shallow, insufficient to bring enough oxygen to the blood to discharge fatigue, which settles in the system.

The Little Things

It is rarely the big things that cause the fundamental disturbances in our nervous system. The average man and woman appears to be able to tap an astounding reserve of energy to face a great emergency. It is the little things that break him down, the small day-by-day trivia that sap his vitality and his energy.

If you have not learned to balance your time budget, you go to sleep at night with an unconscious nagging awareness that you must "hurry up and rest" because there's so much to do to-morrow and so little time in which to do it.

The alarm goes off and the sound startles you into alertness. Your over-night worry about time makes you hustle into your clothes and you discover a spot on your suit you had not noticed. The suit has to go to the cleaner and you must put on something else. It's a minor aggravation but it delays you. In your haste, you gulp your coffee and it burns your throat. You rush towards the door and the telephone rings. You rush back. By now you have to run if you are to catch your usual train. Little things—but you are upset, tense, irritable.

Watch yourself for a day and mark down in your mind all the small disturbances that occur and your own reaction to them. Sitting in your armchair at night—after sitting all day —you are tired, fagged out. Life has a flat taste. You need a lot of rest before you can face to-morrow. "What a day," you sigh.

What little things they were, after all, the irritations that made you "nervous". As a matter of fact, none of them would have mattered if your time budget had allowed you to cope with them or if you had been relaxed enough to see them in their proper perspective.

It is not the amount of work that you do that makes you tired; it is the way you do it.

"We say," William James pointed out, "that so many of our fellow countrymen collapse, and have to be sent abroad to rest their nerves, because they work so hard. I suspect that this is an immense mistake. I suspect that neither the nature nor the amount of our work is accountable for the frequency and severity of our breakdowns, but that their cause lies rather in those absurd feelings of hurry and having no time, in that breathlessness and tension, that anxiety of feature and that solicitude for results, that lack of inner harmony and ease, in short, by which with us the work is so apt to be accompanied, and from which a European who should do the same work would nine times out of ten be free."

Unfortunately, in recent years, the European too has lost, for the most part, his capacity for relaxation. The stresses of war, economic crisis, devastation and fear have thrown his natural rhythm out of balance.

The Way We Do Our Work

Five major mistakes in our approach to our work are:

1. Failure to balance the time budget
We will attempt to change this in the chapter on "How to Live on Twenty-Four Hours a Day".

2. Lack of Organisation
This will be covered in the chapter mentioned above.

3. The impact of confused impressions
This destroys concentration and causes fatigue, and comes from trying to do too many things at once. A quick glance over the headlines on the first page of a newspaper suggests a dozen different ideas to us, each of which leaves a vague impression with a net effect of confusion. The same result comes from a switching of radio dials. This impact of confused impressions results from failure to think things through, to make decisions, to deal with the problems that worry you. The unfinished job and the unfinished problem create residual tensions.

22

4. The impact of training

Please don't be shocked when I tell you that much of our physical, mental, and emotional tension has its root in our early training in good manners. The repression of normal instincts always sets up a tension. We will discuss these later at greater length but let us consider here that virtue instilled in every well-brought-up child—self-control.

What is its effect on your nervous system? You spend the evening with acquaintances and are acutely bored. Boredom creates tension and fatigue but you are too polite to show it. Someone is unexpectedly rude but you have too much control to display your sudden anger. Your boss fires you. You hold your head high and smile.

Each of these situations has created a nervous tension which must be released but you have been taught all your life the "well-mannered" techniques that prevent this release.

5. The misuse of your muscles

Of all factors creating physical tension this is the most common and causes the most widespread havoc to body function. But the cheering note is that these bad habits can be replaced by right habits that will restore proper functioning.

What is the root of this misuse of your muscles? The problem goes back to the transplanting of man from the country to the city, withdrawing him more and more from manual activities and giving him sedentary jobs. The result is a form of life in which he finds it unnecessary to call on many of his muscle groups for any activity, so that in time they atrophy, while at the same time he is made to over-work certain other muscle groups which grow tense and painful and affect the whole body machine.

Transplant a tree to unsuitable soil and in time it will shrink and die. Transplant a man to an environment to which he is maladjusted and his health and his spirits will suffer.

Difference Between Men and Women

I have often been asked whether there is a difference in

regard to tension in men and women. From my experience I would say there is, very definitely.

Tension in man is, very often, a result of being muscle-bound because of an over-development of certain muscle groups, such as the thighs from ball playing, or the deltoid muscles in the upper arm and neck that stiffen up, making the shoulders lose their flexibility and causing shallow chest breathing.

As a consequence many men develop only abdominal breathing, with the result that the intercostals (the muscles between the ribs) become stiff and the lower back muscles become weak. This condition may well be responsible for much of the heart disease that strikes men in their middle years.

The hands of men who do sedentary work are in many cases either too flabby or too stiff, unbalanced in their muscular development and therefore poor in function.

As a rule, men are less likely than women to have deformed feet but more likely to suffer from flat feet. An unexpected but frequent result is sexual difficulties that can be cleared up as soon as they understand the effect of wrong weight distribution on the male organs.

Women who suffer from tension usually have under-developed muscles or atrophied muscles that were never really developed. For this reason, it is generally necessary to awaken nerve sensations that have not been felt before, as a preliminary to putting the muscles to work.

The result of female tension when due to under-developed muscle groups is spasticity—a fixed tension—in the over-strained muscle groups which produces more pain than men suffer from being muscle-bound. This is an advantage because the pain is a warning. Men are seldom aware of their tensions and are therefore exposed to greater danger.

Let's Get to Work

Now that we know what causes tension, we are prepared to

get to work. Our first job is to find out where we are tense and what habits cause that tension; our second job is to master the techniques for releasing tension; our third job is so to plan our lives that we can eliminate tension in the future.

There are people who enjoy ill health, find it an inexhaustible source of conversation, who prefer a good symptom to a cure any day. If you make a point of discussing the things that are wrong with you, the chances are that this book is not for you.

If you genuinely want to feel better and enjoy your own vitality, give each of the techniques a fair trial. Keep at it. They have worked for thousands of others and achieved splendid results. They can work for you. *But only if you work for them.*

This is not a book to be swallowed like a pink pill in the evening in the hope that it will work by itself. It is simply a guide.

And now—let's get to work.

CHAPTER THREE

Head First

HAVE you ever thought of the functioning of your body as you do of the running of your car? In a lifelong study of the body workshop, repairing thousands of worn out backs, legs, shoulders, arms and hands, I have learned that you can do much to make the machine work more smoothly and last longer, without expense for repairs, if you know how to handle it correctly.

By checking the effect of wear and tear on these parts, oiling those that are rusty, tightening those that have come loose, you can give your body machine a complete overhauling so that it will run like new.

The car was all right when you got it, smoothly running and responsive to your demands. But you left it out in blizzards when you should have garaged it, stripped the gears in a moment of carelessness, forgot to oil the parts or keep the brakes in condition or clean the spark plugs. You drove too fast before the motor had a chance to warm up, and the bumper and fenders are misshapen because of unnecessary collisions. You were not paying attention to the way you were driving. Right now there are a lot of rattles. Something came loose when you struck that patch of rough road. The car seems to be on the verge of breaking down.

Well, let's take a look at it because it has to last. You cannot turn it in for a new model. The chances are that you know little about the way it should function, about what it can do for you if you give it a fair chance.

Stand in front of a full-length mirror and look at yourself. Your appearance and the way you feel are a result of the way you have been using that machine. Look at your posture, at the way you carry your head, at the position of your shoulders. Notice the way you stand, the way your feet and legs support you. Now, with a hand mirror, look at yourself from the back. You haven't just one side, like a playing card. Now turn back and look at your face and neck. Are there signs of a double chin? Is your mouth tense? Are your eyes strained? Are you wrinkled? Is there a generally flabby appearance?

The machine looks older and more worn than it should, and far more battered than is justified by the service it has given you. Well, we are going to put it in condition again. If you *want* to feel better, you can learn how to get more work, more energy and more joy out of your body with less fatigue, tension, and wearing out of parts. You can look younger and happier and—with the flowering of your personality—more interesting. But not if it's too much trouble to do anything about it.

The body is a wonderfully constructed and complicated machine. There are 840 muscles. As long as these are kept flexible as a baby's muscles are flexible, all is well with you. But the chances are that some of them are neglected and some are over-worked and strained, with a result in tension, not only causing you pain and discomfort, but often physical illness and mental tension. Those are the muscles we are going to look for now.

Posture and Relaxation

Good alignment, complete breathing, and the kind of general relaxation you get by lying flat on a bed or on the floor are all basic in the work that we are going to do in order to achieve good posture. For, in a sense, good posture, or proper body alignment, is the goal of our work. When it has become functional, you will have achieved relaxation. But there is no sense in talking about posture until the muscles are functioning properly. There is no sense in talking about complete breathing until sensations now dormant are developed in the nose and throat, in the chest and trunk; until you get the

27

feeling of what a really deep breath is like. And certainly there is no sense in telling you just to lie down and relax. If you could do that, you would not be reading this book. You may think you are relaxed if you manage to lie still for a few minutes, although you may simply have replaced nervous jerks with a form of rigidity. Relaxation is a step-by-step process and we'll take each step as we are ready for it.

Using Your Muscles

The chances are that, in this work of overhauling, you will discover far more muscle groups out of condition than you suspected. In reconditioning them, keep in mind that every movement you perform should be done with ease and comfort. When you find that any muscular effort tires you, check the way you do it. Fatigue indicates that you are using the muscle in an improper manner. This applies to all your movements in daily life.

The way you use your muscles in simple, everyday activities will either improve your health or damage it. The right method will keep you in the proper state of balance between normal tension and relaxation. The wrong method will first produce unreleased tension and discomfort and, in the long run, illness.

Every technique that we describe must be read through and understood before you attempt to do it. Wrong muscle use, however diligently practised, can only harm you. In performing any technique you must be familiar with its various phases:

1. Understand the technique and its purpose.

2. Inhale before you make the movement, so that the breath will act as a support for the muscular activity. From now on—not only in learning new habits but in every phase of muscular activity—let your slogan be:

FIRST THE BREATH AND THEN THE MOVEMENT

This conscious breathing becomes automatic before long

because experience will impress upon you that every movement supported by breath is easier to make.

3. The impulse you feel when you start a movement.

4. The carrying through of a movement.

5. The peak of the movement.

6. The relaxation that follows the movement, combined with exhaling.

7. The rest period before a new movement is started.

Head and Neck

Tension lurks in unexpected places. Remember that tension is energy which is blocked instead of being released properly.

To begin with, we are going to see how much tension there is around your jaw. Most people, especially in sedentary work, keep their teeth clamped together and hold their jaw tight. This is a habit of which they are rarely aware but it is apparent to the onlooker because it makes the whole face look tense, strained, older.

How do you set about relaxing that jaw? In the simplest way in the world. By reverting to one of the natural habits which you learned to suppress because you regarded it as a sign of bad manners. I mean yawning. Yawning is nature's release of toxins and waste materials in the blood. It causes a strong downward movement of the diaphragm, pulls in more fresh air and releases the stiffness in the trunk muscles caused by tiredness.

Do you know how to yawn properly? The chances are that you have suppressed so many natural habits that you have lost the sensation that comes with doing them properly.

You may have observed that I frequently use the word "sensation". The healthy, sentient body is a treasure house of pleasurable sensation. The drawing of air into the lungs, the rhythmic movement of arms and legs, the senses of taste and sight, of hearing and smelling and touching, the moments of drowsiness that precede sleep, the normal enjoyment of sex—all these are our normal heritage of sensation.

Less obvious than these, however, and still more important for our health and well-being, is a general sense of suppleness and aliveness in the body. It is this kind of sensation that becomes blunted as a result of the over-use or under-use of various muscle groups. Before trying to restore proper function to the muscles, therefore, we will attempt, by self-massage, to restore sensation to the nerves connected with those muscles. Blunted sensations lead to a feeling of being only half alive. Indeed, the tense person misses not only a sense of well-being but he is depriving himself of the rich emotional life that should and could be his.

Yawning

You start by relaxing your jaw, letting your lower jaw drop loose so that your mouth is slightly open. From now on, keep this in mind and deliberately let your lower jaw drop until your mouth is slightly open whenever you begin to feel strained or tense during the day. If you make it a conscious habit, it will soon become an automatic one. That, by the way, holds good for all the simple, common-sense techniques in this book. For a few weeks you will have to be conscious of your habits but, once learned, they become automatic and will stay with you for life.

Now that you know how it feels to drop your jaw and release that tension around the lower part of your face, you are ready for the next step. With the tips of your fingers massage the area around the hinge of the jaw to stimulate the nerves and get them to function. You will find the right spot in front of the ear. Now let your jaw drop. No, not like that. Don't *push* it, *drop* it. Oh, much farther than that. You stopped when you felt a resistance in your jaws. But you must open wider, much wider. Open until it seems to you that you could take a whole apple in that gaping mouth of yours. Did you hear your jaws crack? Fine. That's just what we are after.

Let your jaw hang open. It will make you feel rather stupid

30

in the beginning. But you have begun to yawn now, an enormous yawn. It seems to you as though you can't stop. You feel it in your eyes, through your head, in your throat and upper chest; the diaphragm lifts, drops again, affecting your lower organs. And while you are not aware of it, that yawn has also helped to improve the circulation to your head.

Really deep yawning is one of nature's best remedies for tiredness and tension. And more than that, it helps to prevent headaches, to save dentist's bills, and to iron out the tension which ages your face.

The loose jaw is a preliminary for good speech and for all good singing. It is essential for proper voice development and helps to prevent over-strain of the larynx for speakers as well as for singers.

Obviously, there are moments when it would be injudicious, to say the least, to do your yawning publicly: say, when your boss is talking to you or you are meeting a new acquaintance, or entertaining a guest. Nevertheless, make deep yawning a frequent habit during the day to release tension, and try it three or four times after you get into bed at night. It's your first step towards combating insomnia.

Your Tongue

The way to relax your tongue is by putting the tip of the tongue lightly behind your lower teeth and holding it there without pressure for a while.

Tongue relaxation is important for the flow of saliva to the stomach, for circulation in the area of the tonsils, for the functioning of the larynx, and for proper tone production.

Your Voice Is You

Although we all know by personal experience how greatly we are affected by other people's speaking voices, millions of us never speak with our best voice because of tense habits acquired in childhood. Few people ever explore the potentialities of their voices. Some are pitched too high or sound harsh; others are stifled as though their owners were afraid to hear the full, clear sound. This is a sign of repression or shyness or inferiority. The tense person, you see, develops a tense voice, and the tense voice can develop tension in the individual.

Voices never lie. You will find it fascinating to observe speech habits and discover how much shyness, hidden fear, and resentment betray themselves through voices. As you become conscious of your own habits and learn to release jaw and tongue, your voice will improve, it will have a better effect on others and you will discover not only that you speak more confidently but that what you have to say will make a far better impression on others.

Your Mouth

Perhaps nothing reveals so quickly your character and your disposition as your mouth: the upcurving happy mouth, the downward discontented mouth, the determined mouth with its lips clamped together like a dog's teeth on the leg of a house-breaker, the compressed mouth of the repressed person, the querulous mouth of the person who "always has something the matter with him".

Several times a day the average woman scrutinises her mouth carefully as she applies lipstick, but she rarely observes one of the first things that other people see about her, its expression.

And what, you ask, has this to do with relaxation? Well, quite a lot. Because a flexible mouth affects not only the impression you make on others but your own well-being. Take the matter of smiling. There is a right way of smiling and a wrong way. The right way not only brings an inevitable response from others but it relaxes you. The wrong way helps to make you tense.

The wrong way is the tight smile, the artificial smile that

barely opens the lips; the smile of the bored person, of the reserved person, of the fatigued committee woman standing in a long reception line.

Take a hand mirror and try this for yourself. The tight smile creates a slight tightness in the chest that you can feel even in your stomach. It is making you tense.

Now try the real smile. If you have drawn into your shell you may find this one more difficult than you expect. This is the open smile. I don't mean that you are to put on the fixed grin of the Cheshire cat. But open your lips, dilate your nostrils, smile until you feel the muscles move over your cheekbones.

What happens? Well, to begin with, this opening of the nostrils lets the air stream into your nose and gives you a buoyant feeling. Your chest widens and you have a sensation of vitality and cheerfulness. And it is contagious.

If you suffer from shyness or repressions, you may feel a trifle foolish the first few times you try it, but keep it up, not only for the sake of the *appearance* of your smile and the flexibility of your mouth and the vast improvement in your expression, but also because, along with the yawning that you are doing, it will begin to awaken new sensations, an awareness of the sheer pleasure of drawing breath into your body.

The chances are that you have so neglected the muscles used in proper smiling that they will be rather stiff and unresponsive at first. Probably you were unconscious of the fact that you have so many muscles in your face and head. Keep using them and your face will acquire more flexibility, more animation, more interest for others.

Because of the constant action and reaction of muscle groups on one another, it is interesting to see the effect of so small a matter as smiling correctly—and once more I mean by that: open lips, smiling until you feel the muscles move over the cheek-bones, nostrils dilated.

1. Your nostrils begin to regain flexibility.
2. Inhaling improves.

33

3. More air gets into your sinuses.
4. You notice a sensation of expansion through your back.

Your Nose

What happens when we inhale with the nostrils drawn?
It requires an effort to get enough air. Many cases of shallow
breathing are due to tense nostrils alone.

Now let the nostrils dilate and breathe with them open. Do
you notice the difference? You get more air into your body
with less effort. What you did not notice was the effect on
your sinuses. Of all the people who have come to me, I
believe the sinus sufferers have been the most grateful. Why?
Because the proper kind of breathing works wonders at clearing your antrums and preventing the common cold. Red,
inflamed eyes are also a frequent result of bad nose breathing
and clear up when the following technique is regularly
practised.

From the standpoint of appearance, the right smile, as
described above, and the proper relaxation of the nose so
that the nostrils are dilated instead of pinched, will do much
to save you a bill for face lifting.

An excellent habit to restore proper function to the nose
is to close the right nostril with your thumb while you breathe
in and out through the left nostril. Now close the left nostril
and repeat.

Close the right nostril with your thumb and inhale with
the left nostril dilated. Close the left nostril with your forefinger and exhale through the right nostril. Do this rapidly
several times and then alternate. If you have obstructions in
your nose, continue this habit, mornings and evenings, every
day. It will clean out the sinuses, shrink swollen mucous
membranes, and help in many headache conditions.

Self-Massage

If you have been a tight smiler and have been accustomed

to breathe through pinched nostrils, it is more than likely that the muscles of your face have become rather inflexible. As a result, there has been a lack of circulation in the surrounding tissue. Each such spot has a tendency to harden because it lacks the circulation that every muscular movement brings to surrounding tissue. This is true, of course, of inactive muscles in any part of the body.

If there is a hardening of tissue around these facial muscles, the nerves in time will lose their perfect connection to the brain, just as a petrol tube that has accumulated dirt will slow down the motor of your car. In the case of your car you have the dirt cleaned out. The same is true of your tissues.

How do you eliminate this hardening and restore circulation? By self-massage.

Stand before a mirror. Take your index fingers and start a slight rotating movement at the lowest point of your nostrils.

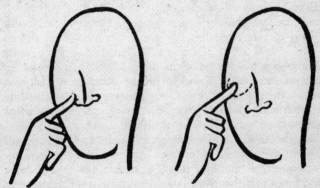

Showing correct position of the finger for nose massage (left) *and sinus massage* (right)

Still using the rotating motion, move the fingers slowly up your cheek beside your nose. The chances are that you will discover several nerve points that are sensitive. Now, still rotating the index finger-tips, move along under your cheek-bones from the nose out to the ear. Now over the cheek-bones, and finally above the cheek-bones.

As your fingers move over this area of your face, it is probable that you will discover that the tissue over the cheek-bones feels more or less hard, as though you were grasping a small round apple. This resistance in the tissue bothered you when you tried to smile broadly. If you keep up this gentle massage over the cheek-bones for several weeks, a few minutes a day, you will restore circulation, leaving the tissue soft and the muscles of the face more flexible.

Now you begin to see why I do not start with techniques for complete breathing. So long as the nerve sensations through the nose are blocked or impaired, your efforts to achieve complete breathing would be fruitless. All of us have far more of these blocked or weak muscular nerve impulses than we suspect. The more of them you can restore, the better you will feel, the better your body will function, and the more vitally alive you will be.

Your Eyes

Your eyes are subjected to more strain than almost any organ of the body. Primitive man looked at distances, at green trees and meadows. Contemporary man uses his eyes for close work, peering for long hours at such minute objects as, for instance, the type on this page, looking down instead of straight ahead or to the side. In some cases, it is possible to guess a person's profession by his eyes—the eyes, for instance, of the hunter or seaman, accustomed to wide vistas.

Only recently have we begun to learn what a staggering proportion of our mental energy is absorbed through our sight. Some authorities claim that it accounts for sixty per cent, some declare that it is as much as eighty per cent. This is an enormous energy expenditure and it is small wonder that much of our fatigue. strain and headache is a result of tired eyes.

The ideal time to check all tension and fatigue is not

36

during the summer vacation or the week-end or even at night after work. The time to check it is when it occurs. Most of you will say promptly that it isn't practical. Yet just as fatigue accumulates as you go through the day, so most fatigue can be checked or prevented then.

Resting the eyes need not be an elaborate matter of lying down in a darkened room. Stop work and look as far away as possible, out of the window at some distant object. Don't stare at it. Look quickly back and forth from a far to a near object, from a large to a small one, letting the eyes shift and relieving the strain on them. Blink several times as you do it. Blinking cleanses the eyes and rests them, besides keeping them moist. If you have been looking at a printed page for a long time, look into the distance and back again, several times, stretching the eye muscles from near to far.

The pioneer work of Dr. Bates on the eyes has indicated that eye-strain is often the cause and not the result of defective vision and that the eye-strain in many cases has its origin in mental strain, or a failure to be completely relaxed.

How to Treat Tired Eyes

The following is the best relaxing technique I have encountered for the eyes:

Drop your eyelids. Do not press them together. Close them lightly. The eyes seem to be moving around under the lids, still tense and staring. Tell yourself that there is nothing to stare at. It is growing dark and there is nothing to see. Very dark. And you are sitting quietly and at ease.

With the tips of your fingers—your eyes still closed—massage your temples gently. Now comes the important part. Imagine that your sight is not at the front of your eyeball, it is at the back. Slowly you feel that your eyes are dropping back into your head until they are in the back of your skull, with the sight on the back of the eyeball so that you are looking back into your head.

After a few moments, open your eyes. They will feel rested

and the tension around them will be gone. This is a practice that should be resorted to whenever the eyes are tired. Make it a habit after you go to bed at night. It is also a great help in preventing headaches due to eye-strain.

This technique can be employed while you are riding back and forth to work and for a couple of minutes every few hours during the day at your desk or while doing household chores. It will not only refresh you but it will make your eyes brighter because it will improve the blood supply.

Your Neck

Feel the muscles of your neck both at the back and sides. If you are a sedentary worker, the chances are that the muscles in the back of your neck are flabby and atrophied from lack of use while those on the sides are strained and tense from overwork.

About eighty out of a hundred persons whom I have examined suffer from pain in the muscles at the back of the neck.

"It's because I work so hard," they declare.

It's actually because they work in the wrong way. The sedentary worker tends to be aware of listlessness and fatigue much sooner than is justified by the amount of work he does. What causes his fatigue is the nerve pressure due to his wrong alignment of vertebræ, resulting in faulty posture. This may interfere with the supply of blood, lymph, and air to the brain.

If you are one of the countless victims of neck pain and fatigue, here is a simple technique to try right now.

Head Lift

Place your hands so that the finger-tips meet at the base of the skull, and *lift hard*, stretching the neck muscles. Do this every half-hour and you will get rid of this annoying pain at the back of the neck.

38

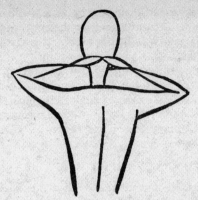

Showing position of hands for the head lift

Small Head Turn

Now let's get to work to limber up those neck muscles, relieve tension, and strengthen the neck so that it is able to hold the head up properly.

Bending over a desk all day, with little change of position, has a tendency to stiffen the neck muscles. The small child has a limber, flexible neck but he soon begins to lose this flexibility. Again the villain of the piece is our old friend Good Manners.

"Don't turn around," the child's mother whispers in church.

"Don't look now," says his friend.

It isn't good manners to turn. And little by little the restraints check natural, instinctive behaviour, the muscles fall into disuse, and the blocked-up energy causes pain and tension.

There are two excellent techniques for limbering up the neck.

The first is the small head turn. The object is to make a circle with your head without moving your neck. Put your hands behind your head so that your fingers touch the first vertebra at the base of the skull. Massage the vertebræ at the base of the skull and at either side with a rotating movement of the fingers. It is from the first vertebra that the head is to turn—*without moving the neck.*

As you start to inhale, turn your chin to the right, up until you feel the stretch under your chin, to the left, and back to the front.

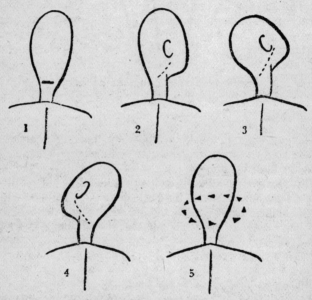

How to turn the head for the small head turn. The broken line is the line of sensation—it shows where you feel the pull. The arrowheads indicate direction in turning.

Now repeat, circling to the left, to avoid dizziness. Try it several times in each direction. Your eyes will be fresher and your scalp will feel more alive.

Pull your chin in firmly and slowly, developing a stretch which will make you feel that your neck is getting longer.

Make this small head turn and neck stretch an hourly habit for a week or so. It is so inconspicuous a gesture that no one will notice it. At the end of that time you will automatically begin to sit with your head more erect. You won't be pulling it up by main force, with that constant, annoying feeling that you should "sit straight". You will be going at it the right way. Get the muscles in condition and posture takes care of itself.

This small head turn makes you less tired, prevents fatigue, teaches you proper alignment of the head, helps you to breathe more deeply, and, as an unexpected dividend, it will prevent a double chin; or, if you already have one, it will gradually go away.

Don't take anything I tell you for granted. Experiment for yourself. I would like to see these words emblazoned:

WANTED—A SCEPTICAL READER

The Big Head Turn

The big head turn is more ambitious than the small head turn. Its purpose is to put in working condition all the muscles that connect the head and shoulders with the trunk. In all my experience I have encountered no one with the exception of a few highly trained professional dancers and athletes who did not have badly aching spots in this region. Doctors are swamped with patients coming for heat treatments to relieve neck and shoulder pains.

The big head turn takes time and concentration to do properly. But once you master it, you will find it an excellent means of clearing out all the bumps and painful tension that have settled around this region.

The chief blood supply to and from your brain is concentrated under the muscle group at the sides of the neck. The more hours you sit, the greater the danger that these muscles will be over-strained and lose flexibility. The tenser they become, the poorer will be the circulation to and from the brain.

41

Sit or stand erect. Drop—do not push—your head so that your chin nearly touches your chest, lower jaw relaxed and hanging loose at the hinges.

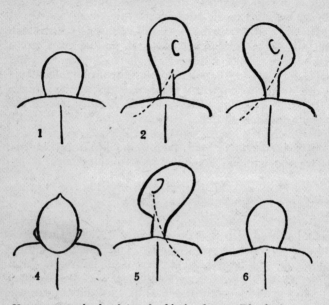

How to turn the head for the big head turn. The broken line shows where you feel the pull.

Now inhale through the nose, and while you continue to inhale, start pulling your head to the right, without lifting the shoulder. You will feel a real tug, which may be rather painful in the muscles of the neck and shoulders. Keep moving the head in a circle until it reaches the centre. Pause for a moment, with the head hanging back, still holding your breath. You should have the feeling that only the muscles at the back of the neck hold the head. The front of the neck is relaxed and without strain, the jaw is loose. This lack of strain over the larynx is important. Now, continue pulling the

42

head around for the rest of the circle, ending with the chin once more nearly touching the chest.

Now slowly pull your shoulder-blades together, which will force you to raise your head and get back in normal position.

Repeat, starting to the left.

If the muscles of your back, shoulders and neck have been functioning improperly for some time you are apt to be sharply aware of their stiffness while doing this exercise. But keep it up whenever your neck gets tired or stiff, and you will discover in the course of a few weeks that the muscles will begin to loosen up, that pain will disappear, and that you can work longer without fatigue.

You will find it restful to make this big head turn after you have been driving your car for any length of time, or after hours in a movie, staring at the screen.

Developing Posture Sensation

And now that you have begun to discover where the soreness and tension are to be found in the region of your head and neck, and to limber up your muscles, you are in better condition for a neck-strengthening technique that is the finest posture builder there is, because it gives you an instinctive feeling for alignment.

Stand with your back to the wall, heels touching the wall, feet straight. Now let your buttocks touch the wall; now your shoulder-blades; now the back of your head. Your arms are against the wall, the palms of the hands towards the wall.

You will feel a strong pull along your spine and up through the vertebræ of your neck. This stretching sensation in the neck is very important. Hold the position for a few moments and feel your breath float through your body like a wave. As you walk away from the wall the sensation of that stretch will remain with you for a long time. If you do this in the morning before going to work and twice a day for a matter of weeks, you will develop an instinct for posture that will stay with you for hours, automatically holding you straighter when you walk or sit down.

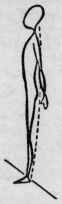

Showing the correct position for standing against the wall

In the beginning it will feel as though a stick were pulling up your neck but that is only an indication of how much those neck muscles of yours need development.

The stronger your neck muscles become, the better the carriage of your head will be, and this is important not only to prevent tension and combat fatigue but also because of its vital effect on your morale and your point of view. I am using the term "point of view" quite literally. Walk with your head down and your eyes peering up. Now hold your head up and look straight ahead. You are aware of an improvement not only in your vision but in the way you feel. Your focus is now proper. By looking at things on a level instead of peering up at them, you have a greater feeling of adequacy. The person who is always looking up at the situation feels that it is too big for him.

Acquiring New Habits

Although you will feel an immediate relief of tension when

you start to apply these techniques for conscious relaxation, you must bear in mind that we are not aiming at alleviating your trouble temporarily. We are aiming at getting rid of tension once and for all. The lasting results show up gradually.

It takes time to change long-fixed habits, particularly when you have been unconscious of many of them. It seems to be a nuisance to be aware of your own habits all the time. In fact, it *is* a nuisance. But keep at it. A few weeks of honest effort to improve the way you feel will bring better dividends in well-being, increased vitality, better looks and better spirits than you would believe.

A Reminder

Make these your new habits:

1. Learn to yawn deeply.
2. Remember to keep your jaw loose.
3. Relax your tongue by resting the tip lightly behind your lower teeth.
4. Smile widely so that the nostrils are dilated and the cheeks flexible.
5. Clean the sinuses by breathing with the thumb and forefinger technique.
6. Massage the tissues along the nose and over the cheekbones.
7. Let the eyes "fall back" in the skull.
8. Shift and blink the eyes frequently during the day.
9. Pull the neck up hard.
10. Do the small head turn.
11. Do the big head turn.
12. Stand against the wall to develop posture instinct, and stretch the neck muscles.

CHAPTER FOUR

As Easy as Breathing

IF you have begun to put into practice the techniques described in Chapter Three, you have awakened nerve sensations through the nose and throat and, by the exercise of your diaphragm in yawning, you have discovered some of the benefits of proper breathing.

Now, before we continue to relax the other muscle groups of the body, let us explore together the vital problem of complete breathing as it affects your ability to relax, your general health, and your mental well-being.

In the *Encyclopædia Britannica*, there is a telling description of the significance of the act of breathing:

"The conception of life is so closely bound up with that of respiration that the very word 'expiration' has come to connote the extinction of life, and 'inspiration' its elevation to a super-human level. Respiration is a process common to all forms of animal life, the reason for which is that the chemical basis of life is essentially an oxydation of tissue."*

A human life actively begins when the first breath is drawn into the lungs; it ends with the final sigh that expels the last breath; it is dependent for its health and well-being, from beginning to end, from moment to moment, on the quantity of oxygen inhaled and the way in which it is inhaled. When the body is deprived of the proper amount of oxygen, it begins to suffer *at once*.

The most obvious example is the breathlessness that comes with choking. The body does not issue some slight warning— as in the case of hunger—that eventually its need for food must be taken care of. It demands oxygen immediately, within a matter of seconds. Otherwise it will die. In less

Encyclopædia Britannica, 1929 edition, article on "Respiration".

dramatic form it shows equally prompt evidence when the conditions are not so acute. Sit bent over a desk for hours without doing complete breathing. Tension settles in the form of aching shoulders, or fatigue is revealed in headache, mental staleness or confusion that hinders your work.

There is no habit in life that pays bigger dividends, and pays them more promptly, than complete breathing. It is the source of your health, your cheerful spirits, your feeling of youth, your energy, and your relaxation.

A healthy baby is the perfect instructor in breathing and relaxation. Watch it and see why. The new-born child uses all the muscles of its trunk that should be involved in the breathing process, those of the abdomen, sides and back. When it cries, one is amazed at the volume of such a little person's voice. How is it possible? Simply because the baby increases the activity of its diaphragm by kicking its legs. The healthy baby has the most relaxed body we know. That is one reason why artists so frequently use it as a model to portray inner happiness.

How We Breathe

When we breathe, the breath enters through the nose. That is why it is important that there should be no obstructions in the nose or in the sinuses. If your child breathes through his mouth, you should have him examined to discover whether there is some malformation or obstruction in the nasal passages.

Mouth breathing is not a satisfactory substitute for nose breathing. Why? Because the nose has the function of an air-conditioning machine. It warms the air in the few seconds that it passes through, raising it to body temperature. It also serves as an air filter, clearing the air of dust particles. This is important because the amount of dirt in the air is appalling.

Passing through the pharynx, air enters your larynx, where your vocal cords open like a valve each time that you inhale so that the air can get into the windpipe, and through the windpipe into the bronchial tubes and thence into the lungs.

Your Lungs and Their Work

The lungs, made up of a spongy, elastic tissue, are cone-shaped organs which fill the greater part of the chest cavity. The right lung consists of three lobes, while the left has only two because the rest of the chest cavity on that side is occupied by the heart.

The function of the lungs is to provide the exchange of gases that we need for living. Tiny blood vessels in the walls of the millions of air sacs of which the lung tissue is composed, receive oxygen from the inhaled air and discard carbon dioxide. Oxygen is the gas that is essential for life. A sufficient amount of oxygen must be taken into your blood to burn up the waste material constantly being formed by the body through the work of all the organs, which act like chemical plants in the system.

In other words, a lack of oxygen caused by shallow breathing means that the waste material in the body is not burned up and the result is fatigue and a lack of zest for living. When your blood is filled with waste materials it gets heavy and lazy and causes poor circulation.

Your Heart and Liver

The lungs are the oxygen tanks of your body while the heart functions as the general pump. The heart sends the blood first through the lungs to pick up oxygen and expel carbon dioxide, returns it to the heart enriched with oxygen and sends it out on a second tour through the opening in the diaphragm called the main artery, into thousands of small tubes that carry the oxygen-enriched blood to all the organs.

On its return trip to the heart, the blood gathers in a most fascinating organ, about which most people know very little —the liver. The liver has five essential functions for keeping us alive, but the only one that interests us here is the purification of the blood after it has been burdened with the waste material of all the organs which it has supplied with fresh blood. The liver lies just below the diaphragm and so you see why the proper function of the diaphragm is so important for your health.

The lungs and the heart fill the whole chest cavity of the body. It is odd that so few people realise that the lungs fill the back as well as the front of this cavity, and extend even farther down in back than in front.

Your Diaphragm Helps Too

The diaphragm forms a kind of partition between the lungs and the other organs of the body, like a movable ceiling. Below it are the stomach, kidneys, intestines, sex organs, and bladder. Therefore, when the diaphragm moves—like a kind of suction cup—with each expansion of the lungs, the organs below it are exposed to a soft pressure which acts as a stimulation. If the breathing is shallow and the diaphragm moves only slightly, all the vital organs that depend for their proper functioning on this stimulation begin to suffer in their own functions. Constipation, stomach, gall-bladder, and kidney trouble are frequently a result of lack of proper function. Therefore, it becomes apparent that complete breathing plays a vital and essential part in our general health, and that its impairment can have widespread results.

Nor are the lower organs the only ones affected by a poorly functioning diaphragm. This muscle plays a large part in assisting the heart with its work. When the diaphragm does little work, the whole burden falls upon the heart, providing yet another reason for the increase of heart trouble. And here we return again to a result of our contemporary living conditions. Nothing makes it more difficult for the diaphragm to keep up its stimulating influence on the inner organs than our sixteen-hour habit of sitting.

But the diaphragm, important as it is, is not the only important muscle involved in breathing. Since the lungs expand

and contract the chest and trunk walls, all the trunk muscles become involved in breathing. And because the muscles of the upper arms and thighs are connected to the trunk, they too are involved to some extent in our breathing. Therefore, whenever any of these muscle groups is under-functioning, it causes a block which interferes with your proper breathing habits, and shallow breathing develops.

Better Breathing, Better Work

Aside from its obvious contribution to the functioning of your organs, to the elimination of waste materials and hence of fatigue, and to the increase of vitality, proper breathing serves another major, and too often ignored, function. It helps the muscles to perform their work.

Try this little experiment. Stand up and lift your arm high, as though you were reaching for something on a high shelf. Now repeat the movement, but as you start to raise your arm, begin to inhale. The second time, instead of lifting the arm, it seemed to swing up with more power and less effort. It felt good because your body was functioning properly. From now on—and for ever, I hope—remember that your watchword is:

FIRST THE BREATH AND THEN THE MOVEMENT.

This is repeated because it is of paramount importance. It applies to all movements, all exercises, all physical activity. *Let your breath work for you.*

The Mind and Breathing

The influence of breathing not only on the body but also on the mind and the emotions has been known to man from the earliest times. That is why the motions prescribed for all religious practices are designed to affect the breathing rhythm. In some cases, the intention has been to accelerate it, in others to retard it.

In some primitive religions, for example, where dancing is

a religious rite, the tempo grows faster and faster to create mounting excitement and finally a trance-like state.

For the Mohammedans, on the other hand, the practice of falling on the ground five times a day with outstretched arms, and feet that have been cooled by bathing, releases all tensions in the body, slows down breathing, and puts the worshipper in a state of mental calm.

The Christian practice of kneeling in prayer with closed eyes and clasped hands also quiets the breathing rhythm, quiets the mind, and prepares one for contemplation.

How *completely* do you breathe? Do you take in a little air so that your upper lung lifts slightly? Or are you aware, as you breathe, that your shoulder muscles move on your back and that the lower ribs expand? Can you feel an expansion in the small of your back? When you have mastered relaxation and proper breathing, you should be able to feel that your breathing lifts the abdominal wall clear down to the pelvis.

No Breathing Exercises

You are not going to study breathing exercises. I have watched innumerable groups of people, young and old, in gymnasiums and singing schools, performing breathing exercises according to all kinds of methods. These poor people breathed to improve their chest expansion, or to cultivate diaphragm or abdominal breathing.

They panted like dogs and they slowed down their breathing like yogis. They breathed before open windows and they breathed lying down. They breathed to a count and they breathed to gramophone records. The harder the poor victims tried, the more damage was done through the partial over-strain of internal organs, while the inevitable outcome was muscular tension.

To understand why there is so much confusion over breathing methods, we must understand the unique position of breathing. The functions of our heart, kidneys and liver, intestines and stomach are all carried on automatically, without

51

our being aware of them, unless pain signals that something is going wrong.

On the other hand, all our conscious movements, such as walking or standing, are controlled by the mind. Before you can lift your arm, you must send a message from the brain to the muscles involved, and the pathways for those messages are your nerves.

Breathing has a unique position. It is the only function that not only works automatically from the moment of birth until the moment of death, but that can also be controlled through the conscious mind. You cannot tell your heart how fast to beat or send a mental order to your liver. But you can impose conscious control over your breathing.

How can you improve your breathing if not by exercises? By paying attention to your daily habits and correcting those which are bad for you. Habits are repeated over and over; in the long run, they make you either healthy or sick, either relaxed or tense, either happy or unhappy.

Breathing is the very root of your life. You may go without food for several days; you won't feel strong but you will survive. You can go without water for many hours. But how long can you go without a breath? Hardly more than a single minute or you will be dead.

Breathing, you see, is vital. Therefore, it is important that you do it properly. How? Not by breathing exercises, but in the only natural and effortless way—according to your own personal rhythm. And that is what we are going to discuss next.

CHAPTER FIVE

Your Own Rhythm

EVERY human being is born with his own personal rhythm, as distinctive and individual as his finger-prints. Whether, as doctors assume, this rhythm is dictated largely by the glands, is unimportant for our purpose. What *is* important is that each human being should learn to be aware of his own rhythm and live in accordance with it.

This personal rhythm is physical, mental, and emotional. When it is thrown off balance, the whole system suffers, mentally and emotionally as well as physically. For the human being cannot be separated into air-tight compartments; a physical body, a mind, the emotions. These three are so inter-related that it is impossible to consider them separately.

The stresses of mechanised life, or our reactions to those stresses, or our reactions to each other—our voluntary attempts to alter our own rhythms to fit those of other people—all tend to make us lose our natural rhythm. And we must regain it if we are to know real health and real peace of mind.

The easiest way in which you can check your own personal rhythm, learn what it is and come to terms with it, is by learning to understand it. Whether you are slow or fast does not matter. What matters is that you yield to the pace that is right for you. Some people breathe slowly, taking an average of only six breaths per minute; others may breathe as fast as twenty-one times per minute. Both types will feel healthy and at ease in their own rhythm; it is right for them.

The Courage to Be Yourself

For some reason, people are apt to regard quickness in itself as a sign of superiority. Quick thinking is taken as a sign of intelligence. A person is apt to pride himself on doing a thing fast. Of course, this is all nonsense. The quick thinker is not necessarily the sound thinker. The person who does things at top speed may not do them well. In the long run, there is no indication that the fast mover goes farther than the slow mover.

What does matter is finding and sticking to your own rhythm. *Have the courage to be yourself*. The phrase is so shopworn, so hackneyed that it seems absurd to utter it, and yet how many people have that essential courage? The moment you disturb your personal rhythm, you harm yourself, physically, mentally, and emotionally.

Take the simplest example of a wrong personal rhythm from the standpoint of timing. Let us suppose that you are naturally a quick-moving person. At some time or other you have taken a long walk with someone who is very young or very old, and as a result you had to alter your own gait and force yourself to a much slower pace. What happened? You came home irritable and tired. But your fatigue was not a result of the energy expended in walking; it was a result of faulty rhythm.

We know the effect on the motor of faulty rhythm and the wrong speed. The dials of motor-cars turn red as a warning when the speed is pushed over fifty miles an hour. The nervous system sends out its warning signals when our rhythms go wrong, but we either ignore the signals or fail to understand what they are telling us.

The more a person lets his own rhythm be his guide, the better he will use his body. This is the secret of grace, and distinguishes such dancers as Pavlova and Markova from the thousands who have acquired dancing techniques by diligent muscle training but have ignored their own personal rhythm. Their movements do not *flow* in the same way; they do not represent the same direct expression of personality.

Our personal rhythm begins with our first breath. So long as it is not upset, we feel well and healthy. It may be upset physically, mentally or emotionally, and the result, so far as

54

our breathing is concerned, will be the same. Illness, pain, fear, sudden shock may any of them upset this rhythm temporarily. Usually we overcome the disturbance without bad after-effects. But if the impaired rhythm becomes a habit, shallow breathing is set up, and we have to learn to regain our old rhythm.

The simplest illustration of impaired rhythm is what we call "losing our breath". We have all done it by running for a bus or train, experienced the gasp and caught breath that accompany the shock of bad news.

A long-range illustration is the common danger of sitting for long hours with bent back. This automatically limits the breathing and establishes a habit which impairs your own rhythm and deprives your system of the necessary oxygen.

Emotions Influence Your Rhythm

All emotions affect this rhythm, joy and happiness can affect it—making us breathe more deeply and expand our chests; grief and sorrow affect it—bowing us over. The phrases, "He is downcast", "he has a heavy heart", have a literal as well as a figurative meaning.

Between these extremes lie all the smaller and less obvious disturbances in our breathing rhythm. A stop for a red traffic light, a reminder that the income tax payment is due, a steak that is tough, Junior hammering on his crib with a rattle, your marriage partner repeating in inexorable detail a story you have heard a dozen times, a political campaign, or a mention of those inflammatory words Capital and Labour—all these can impair your rhythm. The speed and completeness with which you regain your normal rhythm will determine your nervous and mental health.

The moment a baby is quieted after crying, or reassured after a fright, it becomes peaceful and immediately resumes its rhythm. On the other hand, a grown-up will hang on to his tension for hours afterwards, and as a result will be far more fatigued than the baby.

Take some time to-night before going to sleep and start to get acquainted with yourself. Find out what your rhythm really is.

How do you set about finding your own breathing rhythm? Well, *not* by beginning to breathe deeply in a self-conscious manner. That will not teach you anything. The less you do, the quicker and better results you will get. Your job is not to act, not to do voluntary breathing, not to exercise, but simply to *watch and listen to your own body*.

Lie down on your bed in a comfortable position, drop your eyelids lightly, place the tip of your tongue behind your lower teeth.

Now do nothing! You are under no strain at all. The bed is supporting the weight of your body. You are not holding it up.

"Oh, I know how to do that!" you say impatiently. "See, I am resting!" You clamp your jaws together to show your grim determination to relax, you lie still enough, but stillness in itself is not a sign of relaxation. A taut rope may be motionless.

You should observe the person lying on the bed as though it were someone else, someone for whose actions you have no responsibility. Do not try to make yourself breathe, simply watch the way in which you are breathing and what is going on in your body. Don't worry about whether your breath is fast or slow, deep or shallow.

You may observe, and you probably will, that if you lie quietly, there will be a jerky sensation in your diaphragm. This jerking is a nervous habit which millions of people acquire and sometimes it takes a long period of conscious letting go before the jerking stops.

These short, jerking motions do not provide you with enough air and they interfere with the rhythmical functions of your organs. This nervous habit is particularly harmful to the liver and gall bladder. The sooner you acquire the habit of relaxing completely while you lie on your bed, the quicker you will be conscious of a sensation of real peace.

You know that if you want a plant to grow, you cannot interfere by pulling at the roots to see how they are developing. The same goes for the rhythm of your inner organs. Only rest and being let alone can accomplish the desired result. But you will be aware, when the diaphragm quiets down and stops jerking, that your stomach will perform its duties much better because a quiet, deep breath helps the stomach to function through the movement of the diaphragm.

After a few moments, drop your lower jaw *way down* and start a wide yawn. You will notice a downward movement not only above your stomach but extending all the way around to your back.

After yawning several times, lie quiet again, your eyes still closed, imagining that the eyeballs have no sight in front and that they are slipping back in your skull so that the sockets are empty. Do not try to direct your breathing.

After some time you will become aware that your breathing has a certain rhythm; not the one-two—in-and-out—rhythm of breathing exercises; but a three-rhythm; you inhale, you exhale, and you rest. The rest period will vary, sometimes being very brief, sometimes rather long. Whatever that rest period, do not interrupt it and start breathing voluntarily. Wait and remain passive. That rest period is the most important part of the breathing function for the purpose of relaxation. The more passively you wait, doing nothing yourself, watching what goes on inside you, the more quickly you will master the art of relaxation and eliminate nervousness.

In order to develop this passive attitude, you must be alone in a quiet room where you will not be disturbed. If you have no room of your own, wait until your partner is asleep before you start to observe your breathing. In the beginning, you will need the silence and security that come of being alone. In time you will be able to relax whenever you like, even in crowded rooms. This quiet attention to the body can bring such control, even in the badly handicapped—cerebral palsy

57

adults and infantile paralysis victims—that they can sleep in crowded subways going to and from work.

The aim of this whole experiment is to discover what your *unhampered* breathing rhythm actually is. You won't discover it in a moment. If you are tired or keyed up or nervously exhausted or tense or accustomed to shallow and inadequate breathing, it will take time to re-establish your own rhythm. The two important things are: (1) not to try to alter your breathing by any voluntary effort; (2) to achieve so complete a capacity for relaxation that you will *involuntarily* be able to lengthen the pause between exhaling and drawing in the new breath.

How vital this pause is to your well-being has appeared in psychological experiments made during the war when it was discovered that the person whose breathing rhythm had the longest pause was the one least likely to break down under the stress of action. In other words, this *involuntary control*, acquired by relaxation, by doing nothing, pays dividends in increased physical, mental, and emotional stamina under stress. It is the real key to being able "to take it".

Breathing and Relaxation

As you have doubtless observed, this book is based on the idea of inducing the proper breathing, relaxation, body alignment and posture, neither by exercises nor by deliberate corrective techniques of which you are expected to be constantly aware. Human beings, being human, are unable to keep their minds on all their body functions and the way they breathe every moment of the day. Our purpose is to show you what is wrong and how it can be corrected; to point out the things you must watch for during a short period while altering your habits, and then to let the whole process become involuntary and automatic.

Over and over again, I have repeated certain fundamental ideas because they are basic to the subject and their repetition helps to impress them on your memory. Let me repeat, then, that the art of complete breathing is fundamental in your task of acquiring relaxation. Medical experts both in this country and in Europe have been conducting experiments for years and have come to the conclusion that tension can be created by shallow breathing.

Try this for yourself. Take a long, deep breath. What do I mean by a long, deep breath? Well, now that you have awakened breathing sensations through the nostrils and the passages of the head and neck, now that by yawning and the breath that follows it you are aware of the movement of the diaphragm, you begin to get an idea of what a deep breath really is. This is a breath that expands upper and lower lungs, that you feel in your abdomen clear down to the pelvis, in your shoulder and back muscles and in your lower back.

As you exhale, all the muscle groups that—in a baby—are affected by breathing, relax. If your breathing has been shallow, these muscles are unable to relax sufficiently and tension begins to develop in them. If the habit of shallow breathing continues, the muscles of the shoulders and back get out of function, lose their flexibility, and often become as tense as steel. Obviously, the posture is affected and, once the posture is bad, shallow breathing becomes almost a necessity because the inflexible muscles prevent the proper chest expansion. Thus the vicious circle develops.

That is why I said in the beginning that it is pointless to cry, "Stand up straight", until the muscles are in the proper condition. When that is accomplished, your posture difficulties will take care of themselves.

How to Relax

Settle down comfortably on your bed, with garters, braces, belts, brassières and other garments loose, so that there is no binding sensation anywhere.

There is another habit that babies have and that we neglect as we get older. Next to yawning, the best relaxing habit is stretching.

59

Drop you right hand on your right shoulder and swing your right elbow slowly up. Don't simply *lift* it. Take a breath and stretch so that you bring the muscles into play.

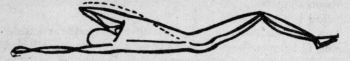

How to do the elbow stretch

You will probably feel an urge to yawn. Give in. Yawn and enjoy it.

Now stretch again, raising your elbow, and notice that the stretch goes clear across your back. It feels good to revive those back muscles that have become lazy. Now drop your left hand on your left shoulder and begin to swing up your elbow. Repeat and feel the stretch across your back, clear below your waist.

Now stretch again and yawn.

This shoulder-elbow stretch strengthens the muscles that get weak from sitting, helps you to stand straight, and releases the tension and fatigue that have settled in your back.

There is a school of thought in regard to the art of relaxation which teaches that to induce the proper body ease in relaxing you must first surround yourself with a multitude of small pillows which are to be placed under the legs, the arms, the head and shoulders at certain strategic angles. Once you have settled yourself in the exact position prescribed for you, you must not move. The next step, according to this method, is to induce relaxation by bringing all your thoughts to bear on the tension of one section of the body after another.

My own experience has indicated that people don't want to be bothered with this array of pillows; that forcing themselves to lie still if they want to move, simply induces more tension, and that breathing and relaxation should be so learned that they become involuntary and *not* voluntary processes. In other words, where relaxation is concerned, I believe in taking it easy.

You know that you are lying on a bed that supports your weight and you don't need a scrap of energy to keep it there. Your body is resting. Because you are aware that the bed does the work, not you, your muscles begin to loosen up, since no effort is demanded of them.

Now let's see how you feel. Your eyes are closed and the sockets feel empty, your tongue rests lightly against the lower teeth, your jaw is relaxed because of your yawning. How about your neck? It isn't supporting the weight of your head. Let it go.

Relaxing the Arms and Legs

Your aim is to make each limb feel as loose as though it had no connection with your trunk. Your best teacher for this complete flexibility is your wrist, which owes its limberness to the constant use you give your hands. Shake your hands up and down while you lie at ease, to remind you of this sensation of flexibility, and then shake the arm to get the same feeling of looseness, first in the elbow and then in the shoulder.

Now start to shake your feet at the ankles just as you shook your hands at your wrists. Stiff, aren't they? Your self-education course in applied relaxation is finished the day that your feet feel just as relaxed in every toe as your hands do in every finger.

Now shake the legs, with a kind of vibrating movement, to get a sense of limberness and looseness in the knees.

Rest again. Let's go back to the quiet breathing, to watching your own rhythm. Rest one hand above the hip so that the fingers lie on the lower abdomen, without pressure. This will help you to observe your own breathing habits.

Complete Breathing

In the beginning of your relaxation practice, you will observe that the expanding movement in the abdomen, as you breathe, starts above the stomach. The better you learn to relax, the lower the starting point of your breathing will be. Complete breathing, when you achieve it, will give you the sensation that your abdomen is lifted from the region between the pelvic bone and the navel. When the lift starts above the navel, it is an indication that your breathing has not yet regained its proper function.

With your hand resting lightly on your lower abdomen, while you are doing nothing but letting the breathing develop by itself; you will observe that the lift in your abdomen will gradually start lower and lower. In all cases of flabby abdominal muscles—a curse particularly of the middle-aged—this new breathing habit brings excellent results because it strengthens the lower abdominal wall and brings a feeling of rejuvenation.

The Experience of Relaxation

When you have learned to lie passively, doing nothing, simply watching your own breathing with detached interest, you will slowly become aware that your body is pervaded by a sensation of calmness; that your harassed feeling of being rushed has slipped away. (WARNING: I say, "When you have learned," because this is not something you can do on the spur of the moment. The fact that you have grasped the idea does not mean that you have achieved the sensation. Relaxation is not something to be read about with the idea that it will work while you sleep; it is something to be experienced.)

The first few minutes are the hardest because you are trying to learn something in a hurry, to find out what it is all about and then rush on to the next thing. That is natural because your trouble is nervous tension. But after you have watched that quiet breathing, and seen that the lift in the abdomen goes lower and lower, that the pause before an inhalation is longer, you will begin to lose your acute awareness of time. When you have really mastered this technique, a few minutes of this complete rest of mind and body will give you a degree of rest which formerly required at least an hour of sleep. Your body will seem like an empty shell through which the oxygen washes like a great wave. Your mind, emptied of sensation, will sink into a kind of Nirvana in which you will hardly be conscious of your surroundings, in which you will almost forget your own name.

This is the state of utter repose—physical, mental and emotional—which the Orientals call meditation. It creates a mood which is an intermediate state between consciousness and sleep, in which you forget your daily troubles.

Generating New Energy

An unexpected benefit of this form of rest is that it enables you to shift in a few seconds to heightened concentration and activity. A few minutes of this rest will restore you completely for new work or for a whole evening after an exhausting day. Few people realise that *the greater the capacity for relaxation, the greater the capacity for action.* Over and over again you will find that the people who have made really prodigious contributions to their world were those who were able to recuperate *as they went along,* so that there was never too great a tax on their energies and so that they were continually generating new energies. The people with enormous nervous energy and tension crack up sooner or later. The hysterical Hitlers break both physically and mentally. Nature is inexorable in performing its executions for failure to obey its laws.

Breathing and Posture

We begin to see that breathing and posture are Siamese twins. One cannot be neglected without affecting the other.

In a sense, as I have pointed out, posture is one goal of our work in relaxation. But I do not believe in developing rules for posture. I have read dozens, hundreds of these rules, and seen the results in the people who follow them meticulously. The result is either stiffness—which is not good posture, for it should be fluid and relaxed—or tension.

What *is* essential is to develop your own instinct for posture.

63

Once you acquire the sensation of rightness and comfort when your body is held correctly—and when you see how much better and younger you look—you will involuntarily strive to regain your proper posture.

The chances are that you lost, or possibly never developed, an instinct for posture, long before the damage became apparent to you, to your family, or to your friends. It may have started when your proud parents urged you to sit up before your muscles were strong enough to hold your weight. (We will talk more about that in the chapter on "How to Prevent Tension in Children".) It may have started when you began to go to school, and sat too long at a desk, or in a chair that was the wrong height or shape, or because you carried heavy school books. Or—if you are a woman—it may have started when, as a self-conscious adolescent girl, you became aware of your breasts and began to walk in a slumped position to conceal them—a common condition.

What is Posture?

There is more nonsense talked about posture than about almost any subject with the possible exception of politics. It has been going on for a long time now—a couple of thousand years or more—and, to judge by the results, the advice is getting worse and worse.

Look at the Greek statue of the discus thrower and see the beautiful balance, the flawless weight distribution, the rhythmic beauty which is the result of a man's personal rhythm and his sense of body alignment at their perfection.

Then picture a line of marching German soldiers, with their ramrod stiffness, their ugliness of movement, their muscular tensions.

The gymnastic exercises which are the foundation of practically all physical training to-day developed in Prussia after Napoleon conquered the Germans. Its purpose in the beginning was to whip untrained and uneducated farm boys into tractable soldiers in the shortest possible time—and it worked. The rigidity and tensions which it developed tended to produce the most admirable obedience because they destroyed much of a person's self-confidence or feeling for his own personality. Automatically he became a "yes man".

Try it for yourself. Stand rigidly erect, head stiff, arms and legs stiff, shoulders back, stomach pulled tightly in. Now, while you hold this position, imagine that someone is lunging at you. Can you fight back or protect yourself? Of course not. But it's a fine position in which to take orders.

Over the course of the years, the gymnastic methods have been modernised and modified but they are still not wholly satisfactory because the accent is on muscle development rather than on flexibility.

Posture is not the achievement of a ramrod position. Posture is not stiffness, it is relaxation. It is not tension, it is control. Posture does not mean simply the straightening out of the body; it means primarily the proper alignment of the body. When the body is properly aligned, your movements will have a sense of harmony.

Anyone can acquire a good posture if he will take the trouble to find out which muscles are functioning wrongly. And posture, you see, comes not through rigorous exercise, but through relaxation. By taking it easy.

"As easy as breathing," people say. Well, see how breathing affects your posture. Not merely by its effect in releasing tense muscle groups but by helping you acquire that posture so dear to the hearts of the gym teachers—"straightening up". Take a slow, deep breath. What happens? As your lungs fill with air, they expand. To make room for them, you are forced to lift your chest. Then what? As the chest goes out, the stomach comes in. The proper breath, in short, did without effort what you have been trying to achieve by throwing back your shoulders before you made them flexible enough to carry their share of the burden.

It becomes increasingly apparent that Voltaire was right when he said, "A good deal of human illness could be cured by breathing."

Much of mental illness is a result of lack of harmony between feeling and thinking. The mind loses control because an emotion such as unhappiness or loneliness or fear has been too overpowering; or because, in an attempt to escape from these realities, people withdraw so far into a world of fantasies that they cross the border of insanity. One of nature's best regulating forces for the balance of mind and emotions is the process of physical breathing.

Imagine, for instance, that the telephone rings and someone informs you that a dear friend has just been killed in an accident. The shock stops your breath; the breathing rhythm is completely disrupted. Even after the first tension is released around the chest, your breathing will be shallow and irregular. At length, nature—maintaining its marvellous balance between mind and body—makes you give a deep sigh which brings relief.

A sigh is a strong exhalation which forces the muscles to relax completely, but while it relaxes you, it leaves you with a feeling of sadness and physical depletion because the oxygen has been expelled from the lungs. But in a few seconds, your lungs will demand air and you will take a deep breath to compensate for that sigh. The lungs will expand, you will feel this expansion not only in your chest but in your back. And with this first long breath, you will start to regain your composure and be able to think clearly about what must be done.

The effect of proper breathing on the mind is incalculable. It affords not only clearer thinking but better concentration. Only the relaxed nervous system can exploit to the full its innate potentialities. The relaxed person is best equipped to absorb new ideas.

This fact, incidentally, was said to be the source of much of the late President Franklin Delano Roosevelt's strength in persuasion. He had an exceptional capacity for relaxation and, because he was relaxed, he was able to induce relaxation in those who talked to him. *Only the relaxed mind is open to ideas;* it is almost impossible to succeed in persuading or changing the viewpoint of the tense person. Because the person to whom he talked was relaxed, it was possible for the President to carry conviction. Many people who entered his office in a hostile mood and left it in a co-operative spirit attributed the result to the President's charm. In a majority of cases, it was merely that he was a master of relaxation.

This fact has a staggering pedagogical significance. Teachers who are able to produce relaxation instead of tension in their pupils are amazed by the improvement in their work. In every case, grades go up and the child's approach to his work is different, keener, more alert.

Another phase of this mind-body relationship is that, by regaining control of the muscles through relaxation, and thus in turn of the mind, you find a most important improvement. You learn to control your feelings. Many of the appalling number of crack-ups that occur to-day, over-crowding the mental hospitals, are a result of failure to teach our children the basic unity of mind, body, and emotions, and of the preponderant effect of correct breathing on all three.

CHAPTER SIX

Relief for Aching Hands, Arms and Shoulders

W E have interrupted our check-up on the wear and tear of your muscle groups to discuss the importance of breathing because the proper use of your breath is so important in restoring right function to your body. Let me repeat again that henceforth, not merely in trying out these new corrective habits, but in all your motions in daily life, apply the rule: FIRST THE BREATH AND THEN THE MOTION. This cannot be stressed too strongly.

About ninety-five people out of a hundred feel more or less pain in the muscles that run along the top of their shoulders. By the end of the day the shoulders are sore and uncomfortable.

This is largely an occupational pain brought about by the conditions of modern life and the lack of those stretching movements, such as pitching hay or old-fashioned domestic labours like hanging up sheets. These actions require upswinging movements that act as a counter-balance to sedentary man's usual movements, which entail clasping or carrying things.

If you stop to analyse the routine movements with which you use hands, arms, and shoulders, you will realise that, for the most part, they involve bent fingers and a drawing of the upper arms close to the body. It is rare for us to stretch our hands and push the arms away from the body with a free, swinging motion. As a result, certain muscle groups in the arms and shoulders get almost no use while others are overburdened. These are the ones that you feel aching when you touch the tops of your shoulders.

The chances are that you have spent time and money for heat treatments and other remedies with only partial or temporary relief—yet you can get rid of these pains completely by learning the proper use of these muscles. Before doing this, however, we must examine the muscles in the forearm, the hand, and the fingers, because much of the discomfort in your shoulders is caused by the misuse of your hands and arms.

Your Hands

Let us start by examining your hands. The diagram (see page 70) shows you the points that you should consider, as these are the ones most frequently affected by unreleased tension.

One culprit that gives people far more trouble than they ever suspect is the thumb. Feel the spot marked A on the diagram. Is the tissue between the thumb and the hand soft and relaxed? The chances are that it is stiff, hard and rigid. This means that neither the hand nor the arm are getting the proper nourishment because circulation is impaired. Massage, particularly of this muscle on the left thumb, will not only rest the hand and improve the circulation of the arm, but it will even cause a sensation of relief in the region around the heart, because these nerves are connected with the nerves of the circulatory system.

Massage this tissue with a rotating movement of thumb and forefinger. Do not be afraid to exert quite a lot of pressure, but stop for a few days if it hurts badly. After you have worked away at this for a few days or a few weeks, depending on the degree of tension, you will be aware of a sense of relaxation through your whole hand.

Another possible stiff spot is the area marked B on the diagram. This too should be given a firm massage, followed by swinging the thumb around in a wide circle to limber it up.

NOTE. In discussing techniques for relieving muscle tension, I do not say, "Do this for so many minutes," or "Continue for so many days or weeks." You yourself will be aware of the amount of time the various muscle groups need for relief. And the cheering point to bear in mind is that when you have once relieved the tension, the relaxed condition will remain with you. Proper function will take care of it in the future.

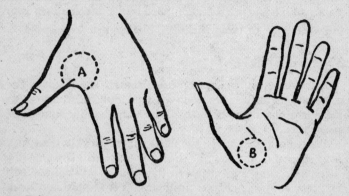

Points to massage on the hand for relief from strain and tension

Stiff and Swollen Finger Joints

When you have finished with your thumb, take a look at the other fingers. A cause of discomfort for a great many people is the first joint just below the finger-nail. At this point the skin tends to get shrivelled and to look shiny. If pain, swelling or stiffness develop, people are afraid to move their fingers, and therefore increase the stiffness by lack of use.

Start at this top joint and massage with the thumb and forefinger of the other hand. Use a good firm movement, so that you really feel the pressure around the joint. Bend the finger up and down. Frequently this shrivelling is just a result of writing or other work that forces you to hold your fingers in a bent position without ever really stretching or relaxing them. It may take some weeks before the tissue below the skin loosens up. But stop to think how long it took for it to become tense and stiff in the first place.

By increasing the flexibility and relaxation of your finger-tips you will improve your ability to do things. If you play the piano, your tone will sound better; if you sew, the work will progress more quickly. Writing will be easier and your handwriting will have more freedom. In normal everyday life nearly all our movements bend our fingers inward—grasping something, carrying packages, holding a fork or spoon.

Relief for Back of Hand

Now what about the back of your hands as a result of the constant pull of the muscles in only one direction? The same thing happens to the back of the hand that happens to every other part of the body where one set of muscles is over-

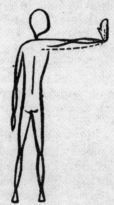

Correct position for obtaining relief for back of the hand

worked and another set is under-worked. It grows stiff.

Stand at arm's length from the wall with your arms out-stretched and the palms of your hands flat against the wall, fingers extended, wrists bent so that the arms are at a right-angle with the hand. Try each hand separately or both together.

You didn't know that these muscles were so stiff, did you?

71

That is natural, however, when you consider how long they have been out of practice. You feel the pull at your elbows and in your upper arms as well as in the wrist and on the back of the hand. Try this movement several times a day until you have re-learned how to stretch your fingers and bring into play those neglected muscles on the back of your hand and in your wrist. This will also help you to develop your forearm muscles.

Bend the fingers of each hand back as far as they will go several times. After a few weeks you will discover that the swollen, or shrivelled, joints are getting normal again, that the hands feel limber and rested, that the shoulders are giving you much less trouble, and—as an extra dividend—that the appearance of your hands has improved and circulation is restored to normal.

A pianist came to me for help after she had tried all the well-known heat treatments for shoulder pains that prevented her from playing.

Rest was prescribed by her physician and when she resumed playing, after some weeks, a numbness had developed in her fourth finger. The tissue in the first joint of this finger felt dried out and as stiff as leather. I started to loosen up the joint by a rotating massage and moved the joint around for greater flexibility.

At first there was a great deal of resistance, but as soon as the joint regained its proper function of bending and stretching, the numbness disappeared and so did the shoulder pain. In her case, and in so many others, we cannot tell whether the root of the trouble lies in the finger joint or in the shoulder. Experience shows only that there is a close connection, and that, in the case of shoulder and arm pains, it is always important to examine each finger as a potential source of the tension.

After you have massaged the thumb and finger-joints and stretched those tight muscles on the back of your hands, stretching the fingers backward, shake your hands up and down hard at the wrist. This limbers up the wrist and relaxes the entire hand.

72

If you continue patiently with this re-education of the hand muscles until the joints become flexible again, I promise you that you will neither suffer from cold hands in winter nor from the discomfort of stiffness that, in many cases, is mistaken for rheumatism. Even the swellings around the joints will disappear in time. For all musicians and typists this capacity for hand relaxation will prove to be an inestimable boon.

Writers' Cramp

In case of writers' cramp, or pain in the forearm, the trouble may well lie in the tense muscle between the thumb and the hand, for which treatment has just been recommended.

However, there is another villain in the case, which is frequently a mental rather than a physical block. A typical example of the psychological reasons for writers' cramp appears in the following case.

A refugee from Europe had to leave her beloved mother behind under Hitler's regime. On board the ship that brought her to the United States she started to write a letter to her mother. Suddenly a pain developed in her right arm and became so acute that she could no longer hold the pen. For over two years she was unable to write because of the cramp that developed in her muscles. What happened was that when she began to write to her mother she was conscious of overpowering fear for her mother's safety, which, with her own sense of guilt over her escape, brought about the muscular tension. The hand began to stiffen and before long the habit had become fixed. It took a long period of patient effort to relax the muscles and restore the proper function.

Your Arms

Examine your forearm, resting it on the table. Is it just a flat bone covered with skin or is it round and equipped with functioning muscles? Now, with your forearm still resting on the table, raise your hand. If the forearm muscle is working properly, you will pull your hand up at the wrist by means of the muscles on top of the arm. If it is under-developed, you will have to push the hand up with the under-arm muscles. That is, you will have to call on the wrong muscles to perform the action because the right ones are not in working condition.

For example, the typist whose arm muscles are under-developed presses too hard with her finger-tips, and this over-use of the wrong muscles not only inflames the nerves of the shoulders but affects her chest flexibility and, indirectly, her heart. So the time spent in developing these under-arm muscles will not only make her feel better but stave off what, in time, might become a serious difficulty.

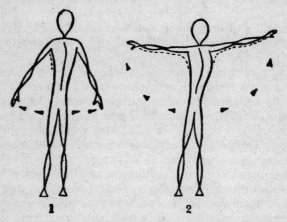

1   **2**

Showing how to do the arm stretch. The broken line indicates where you feel the sensation—the arrowheads show direction.

Arm Stretch

Stand at ease with your feet about six inches apart. As you inhale, lift your arms to the side, palms down.

The inhalation makes the ribs under your armpits expand,

74

and this expansion in turn helps to force your arms to swing up. You feel as though the arm is being lifted effortlessly. As you do this, try to imagine that you are imitating a bird, and indeed, the sensation, as chest and arms rise, is not unlike that of soaring.

Now try the same arm stretch without inhaling. You will see that this causes a muscular strain in the upper arm and feels unpleasant, while the one which you performed with the breath was devoid of strain.

Repeat this arm stretch, inhaling first, and when your arms are out at shoulder level, stretch your third and fourth fingers until you feel the pull all through the hand. At the same time keep the thumb and index finger relaxed. This stretching of the fingers makes you feel as though a wire were pulling from the finger-tip to the arm-pit and this sensation gives you a feeling for the right alignment of the arm.

How the Arm Stretch Helps You

After reading this paragraph, try the arm stretch once more. The longer you hold it, the more you will become aware of how the muscles of your upper arm and shoulder work together, how your neck relaxes and how your upper chest expands.

This position gives you an instinct for proper body alignment, and this physical harmony helps you to regain mental and emotional self-control when you feel "all mixed up".

The arm stretch will help to make you warm and comfortable when you feel creeping over your back the disagreeable chill that precedes a cold. It will also develop the triceps and help you to overcome flabby upper arms that prevent you from wearing sleeveless dresses. This is the best method for improving the looks of the upper arm and its effect on posture can be noticed for hours afterwards, and you will unconsciously straighten up while you sit and work.

You must always keep in mind that it is not the moment of concentrating on your movements alone that brings you

75

..., *no matter how good it may feel at the*
... *newly aroused nerve sensation that stimulates*
... *muscles to participate in work that helps to increase your*
vitality and buoyancy.

If you make it a habit to do this arm stretch for one minute every morning before breakfast, the reminder of this stretch will last for hours and prevent you from slouching while sitting at work.

Why does the arm stretch have so much effect on posture? There is a big muscle in your back called the latissimus dorsi and it is involved in every arm lift you perform, *when you inhale*. If you lift your arm without taking a breath, or if you are a shallow breather, the muscle does not participate in the movement, nor do all the layers of muscle that lie below it. Because you deprive it of the proper use and make it lose its flexibility, you damage your back, as this is one of the strong back muscles that hold you up. Every inhalation expands the back and through this expansion the latissimus and the other muscle layers below it take part in the movement.

Watch your use of your arms for the next few days in your simple, routine movements. Observe the misuse you have been giving them. Learn to profit by this arm swing, each time with a breath, in daily habits. Sooner than you expect, the proper habit will become automatic. For instance, men should be conscious of the arm swing when shaving. Women should use the arm swing in brushing their hair, or reaching for something from the kitchen shelf, or making beds and spreading sheets.

Don't Cross Your Arms

By the way, have you developed a habit of sitting with your arms crossed or tightly folded over your chest as though hugging yourself? Have you ever noticed what this does to you?

1. It pulls your shoulder-blades out of place.

2. It gives you a round back.

3. It blocks your breathing and makes it shallow.

When you find yourself standing or sitting with crossed arms, let them drop to your side.

Your Shoulders

Thousands of people who have pains in and around their shoulders live with the idea that they have rheumatism or arthritis and that not much can be done to rid themselves of their nagging pains. To avoid discomfort, they use their arms as little as possible, and in turn their troubles grow.

In hundreds of cases where the sufferers have diagnosed their own trouble as arthritis or rheumatism, or even when these conditions have actually developed, it has been possible to restore proper muscular function and get rid of these pains. How often they prove to be due to wrong muscular function, to weak and under-developed under-arm muscles that force you to use the wrong pressure on your fingers, or to poor breathing that fails to expand your chest and make the shoulder and back muscles flexible, or to the strain and tension that come from not knowing how to lift.

Relieving Tension in Shoulder Muscles

Before going farther, let's stop right now and get some relief for the tension in those shoulder muscles. How? By reverting to your healthy baby instinct—stretching.

Try it now. Inhaling slowly, lift your arms to shoulder height, with elbows bent and finger-tips resting on your shoulders.

Raise the left arm with a firm, pulling motion, as far as it will go. Don't just lift it up. There's no benefit in that. Pull it up so strongly that you can feel the pull through your shoulders and down your back. And while you are inhaling, by the way, don't try to pull in one long, gasping breath.

77

Inhale in a series of short, quick breaths as though breathing the scent of a flower. Then exhale. Repeat this stretch with the other arm.

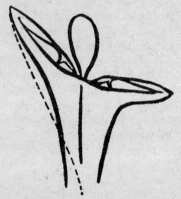

How to do the standing elbow stretch

Now, as an experiment, try this stretch without inhaling. You see, the stretch does nothing at all for you unless you inhale.

How far-reaching the effect of muscular use and misuse can be is illustrated in the case of Miss McLeod, who is a waitress. She came to me, complaining of severe headaches that began about two hours after she started work. The usual cure for that is to have the eyes examined for glasses or to take an aspirin. But our job was to study the way in which she did her work.

I asked her to show me how she carried her tray and I saw at once that she tensed her back muscles and cramped her upper arm and shoulder.

"Why," I asked, "are you so tense when you work?"

Miss McLeod stopped to think and said that it was because of the hostess, of whom she was afraid. In order to please the hostess, she was constantly in a hurry. The combination of tenseness and hurrying made her breathe too fast. The shallow and impaired breathing were beginning to develop a nervous heart. She was holding her breath too long through fear. The back muscles and those of the upper arm were cramped and circulation to the head was cut off. Hence the headaches. But Miss McLeod's trouble was not merely the headaches; she was suffering as well from physical and mental tension, and the poor function which resulted could easily lead to heart trouble.

The first thing, I explained, was to learn how to use her body properly so it would not wear out. Those headaches were like the red dial on the speedometer. They showed her that she was going too fast. The next thing was to learn how to take it easy, how to relax her muscles so that she would have less body strain; with the strain released, she would lose her fear. And with the loss of her fear, the attitude of the hostess would change towards her.

And the important part of all this for Miss McLeod was to learn how to re-train her muscles for right functioning. In other words, she had to learn *how to lift*.

How to Lift

Before you lift, start to inhale. The expansion under the armpit almost forces you to lift your arm. The arm lift becomes an arm swing, and the shoulder muscles co-operate instead of taking the full burden. The result of this changed habit will be improved posture, a strengthening of your back muscles clear down to the waist-line, and a great relief of shoulder tension and pains.

This arm lift is a protection in all industrial work which requires lifting. It protects you from straining your back, which is one of the most frequent and severe of all occupational injuries.

Bras, Shoulder-Straps, and Braces

Another unsuspected source of shoulder pains in women is

the wrong kind of straps on bras. Stout girls with a heavy bust are prone to select tight bras with tight straps in order to make their bust appear smaller. Frequently the straps are so tight that the skin on the shoulders becomes red and shoulder pains follow.

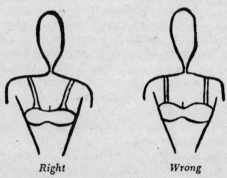

Right   Wrong

Showing the correct, slightly diagonal position of shoulder straps and incorrect, taut position

Here are three points to bear in mind in selecting a bra:

1. Always try it on while you inhale. Then you will be sure that you have room enough for a deep breath. A tight bra will restrict your breathing and develop shallow breathing habits. This shallow breathing in turn may be the cause of tense intercostals (the muscles between your ribs) and a very sensitive area around the breast bone, as well as of many internal troubles that develop in later years.

2. Choose a bra that fits you comfortably and into which you do not have to force your bust with a resulting pressure. The breast is a delicate organ with many glands and every kind of pressure should be avoided. With the increase in breast cancer, women are beginning to learn of the danger from injuries and heavy bruises. The painful constriction of too tight a bra is also dangerous.

3. Consider your shoulder-straps. If they are too far out on the shoulder, you feel that they are slipping, and this sensation forces you to make awkward movements many times a day to keep them up, makes you tense and creates shoulder pains.

The straps should always have a piece of elastic at the end, at least two inches in length and fairly wide, so as to distribute weight and not concentrate it in one spot. The elastic allows expansion and enables you to breathe deeply. Frequently, tight shoulder-straps develop knots or ridges on the shoulder. Countless treatments of diathermy, heat, and massage could be eliminated if you would use a little forethought in selecting shoulder-straps and properly fitting bras.

If you have already developed impaired breathing habits from wearing the wrong kind of bra, you cannot expect that your breathing will immediately return to normal or that your shoulder pains will stop at once, particularly if you have acquired the lumps that seventy-five out of every hundred women have along the top of their shoulders.

Self-Massage for Shoulders

You can speed your own recovery by self-massage. Start at the base of the neck and, with a rotating motion, massage the top of the shoulder. Where you find sore spots, continue the massage until tension relaxes and circulation improves.

Finish this massage by rubbing down from the first vertebra just below the base of the skull to the base of the neck and you will feel a wonderful sensation of relief.

Men's braces are another cause of shoulder pains because they are frequently worn so tight that they encourage inflexibility in the chest muscles with consequent shallow chest breathing.

Business men who are burdened with heavy responsibilities require great muscular flexibility to enable them to throw off fatigue and get the necessary relaxation. The binding of tight braces and belts is injurious in the long run and is the easiest thing in the world to remedy.

Shoulder Rolling

A wonderful help in restoring good breathing habits, because it makes the shoulders and upper chest flexible, is shoulder rolling. Once you acquire this flexibility your shoulder pains will really be gone and stay away for ever.

Lift the shoulders as high as they will go and then pull them forward, down, back and up again. Be sure that you make a complete circle.

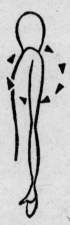

How to do the shoulder roll

Now reverse the movement, beginning the movement by swinging back and down instead of forward and up, so that you feel the shoulder-blades move easily across your back.

Shoulder Flexibility

The shoulder-blades, called scapulæ in medical terms, are

82

two flat bones that cover the back from the second to the seventh ribs. These bones are held in place by muscles and are not connected to the spine; but the upper end of the shoulder-blades, together with the clavicle, form the glenoid cavity into which the humerus—the bone of the upper arm—fits. This connection with the arm explains why all arm movements more or less involve the flexibility of your shoulder.

For the most part, the strong muscles of the shoulders get far less activity than they should have to keep them flexible. Therefore, although I promised that this book would not give you routine drills to do, there are a few motions that you must do for some time in order to limber up these stiff muscles.

Two Arm Swings

Flexibility of stiff shoulder-blade muscles is best achieved through arm swings. Don't approach these arm swings as though you were drearily forcing yourself to do some distasteful exercises. You cannot get a sense of proper body alignment or of your own personal rhythm in that way. As the arms swing forward, try to imagine that you are imitating the motions of a bird; get a sensation of soaring flight.

1. Bring your hands together, back to back, thumbs down. Keep your elbows straight. As you start to inhale, swing your arms forward, up, back, and down. (See page 84.)

When you start to bring your arms down from the swing, you will feel a resistance in the shoulders which is the reason for the whole swing. Leave your shoulder-blades quite loose and feel them glide towards the spine until they touch. It is this soft gliding movement across the back, while you swing your arms down and exhale, that brings you the real benefit.

In the beginning, you will be stiff and probably discouraged, but if you keep up this swing for some weeks you will enjoy it. It will keep out all tension from your neck and back.

2. With your arms hanging at your side, palms out, start to swing them back and up in a circle.

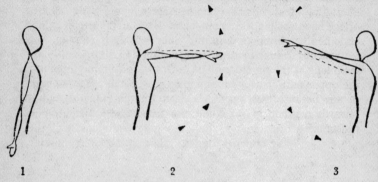

1   2   3

How to do the first arm swing

Here your difficulty is at the start. If you feel very stiff, try one arm at a time. Do it in front of a mirror so that you can make sure you neither turn nor bend your trunk. Only the arms should make the swing. The shoulder-blade muscles may be too stiff or too weak in the beginning to work easily, but do not give up. These swings are an important step in improving your posture and in achieving the self-confident appearance that gives other people confidence in you.

The results of really keeping at these two arm swings over a period of a few weeks are truly amazing. My pupils invariably report that they are asked: "What makes you look so much taller? I've never seen you look so well. Have you been losing weight? You look like a different person. Have you just heard some good news?" This reaction has become so unfailing that I now prepare my pupils for it in advance and they are greatly amused when it happens.

But you accomplish more than this improved appearance by working for shoulder flexibility. You discover that your shoulder-blades really act as a support, something that you

84

can lean on like the back of a chair. When you lean on your shoulder-blades, feeling how they support your back, your stomach and abdomen move too; pulled in not by a conscious effort that creates tension but because of the proper function of the shoulder-blades. Your chest lifts and the stomach and abdomen are lifted as a result; your neck feels relaxed, able to turn in all directions without tension and strain.

So long as the shoulder-blade muscles are stiff and inflexible, the upper part of your lungs is deprived of the proper amount of air, because it is too much effort for the lungs to expand towards a group of inflexible muscles that set up a wall of resistance.

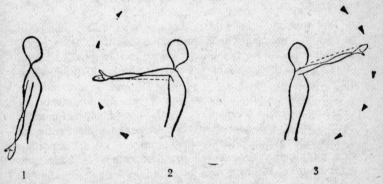

1   2   3

How to do the second arm swing

Double Chin

One unexpected result of shoulder and neck flexibility comes with the disappearance of the double chin, which is a secret source of worry and unhappiness for many middle-aged women. No beauty-parlour treatment can accomplish for you the work of rejuvenation that comes with this type of flexibility. It rejuvenates. The double chin disappears. The wrinkles in the neck disappear.

Mrs. Thomas was a public speaker. She developed a double

chin and dreaded returning to the lecture platform in the autumn because she not only looked much older but she had lost her attractive appearance. She tried everything anyone recommended: a chin-strap at night, creams, massages. But the double chin was still there.

I started her on arm swings and shoulder flexibility exercises and showed her how to massage the neck muscles which had grown tense with strain.

Three months later she went on her next lecture tour and wrote to me in high spirits. The knowledge that her features were restored and her appearance had regained its former youth and attractiveness gave her poise, and the absence of fear of criticism of her looks freed her energy and brought quick response from her audience.

"We women," she wrote, "know what a double chin can do to make us inefficient." And she added that, as an extra dividend, her voice not only sounded better as a result of relaxing her throat muscles, but that she could talk longer without getting tired.

And while we are on the subject of personal appearance— and who is really indifferent to it?—how about improving those hollows you have developed from round shoulders, so that you can wear off-the-shoulder dresses? Try the shoulder swings for some weeks and all your clothes will look better on you because of the improved shoulder line.

These arm swings also help to relieve another curse of the middle-aged, and that is the dowager's hump on the back of the neck. I have seen so many of the humps on the back of the neck vanish as a result of these exercises that I warn my classes in advance that I won't be responsible for tailors' bills.

What happens is that the flexible shoulders massage your fat at this point each time you move them, and the spot that got deformed because it was deprived of proper function loses these masses of fat. Therefore, you need not fear that the dowager's hump will return. Because, even if you never exercise, the right habit of using your shoulder-blades as you inhale will prevent the fat from settling there.

A Reminder:

1. Keep your hands flexible by:
   Massaging thumb and finger-tips.
   Stretching the back of the hand and bending fingers backward.
   Shaking hands at wrist to keep them limber.
2. Do arm stretch to develop under-arm muscles and get a sense of body alignment.
3. Do not cross your arms.
4. Do the elbow-shoulder stretch.
5. Inhale before you lift.
6. Choose the proper bras or braces.
7. Practise shoulder rolling.
8. Limber up shoulder muscles by arm swings.

CHAPTER SEVEN

Help for Your Feet

THE New York *Times* once published a little article saying that far more divorces were due to foot trouble than people ever realised, because people with aching feet are unpleasant without being aware of it. We all know what a toothache means, but we rarely make allowances for the agonies of people who suffer from aching feet. Nor do we ask, in cases of internal organic trouble, whether the feet ache often and tension is a result of poorly functioning feet. In such cases, the internal trouble will never really be cured until the feet function properly.

Referred Pain

My experience has shown over and over again that, when people come to me complaining about pain, it is necessary to look for the real root of the complaint which, as often as not, is at a faraway spot—and very often indeed in the feet.

Examples of referred pain are nowhere as common as they are in the case of foot troubles, perhaps because an overwhelming proportion of people have badly functioning feet, as was revealed during the last war. Pressure on the sensitive nerve endings in the feet often causes headache, muscular tensions and even sinus trouble!

The head nurse at a children's hospital complained for some time about pain in her knee. It became so severe that she was afraid she would have to give up her job, which required a great deal of standing and stair-climbing.

Doctors X-rayed her several times and tried every remedy but they were able neither to relieve her pain nor to find the cause.

When she finally came to me in despair I did not examine her knee. Instead, I examined her feet and there I found what I thought might be the root of her trouble. The outside of the foot was under-functioning, and there was stiffness and lack of flexibility from the fourth and fifth toes through the foot to the ankle joint and all through the leg; while there were over-strained muscles and ligaments at the inside of the foot, especially around the big toe and the inner arch.

Relaxation treatments and re-education in the proper use of the foot brought complete relief in a few weeks and she was able to return to work. As long as I could follow up the case, there had been no recurrence of the pain in her knee.

Let's look at another case. Mrs. Adams, a housewife, was a victim of splitting headaches which came on after her shopping trips, and she had become a good customer for aspirin at her local chemist.

After listening to her complaints I asked her to remove her shoes and stockings.

"But," she protested, "my trouble is headaches!"

"I know," I agreed, "but perhaps your headaches are caused by your feet."

As she walked in, I had observed her badly shaped legs and realised that neither legs nor feet functioned properly. Obviously, the function would be worse when she was loaded with heavy bundles of groceries.

On examining her feet, I found that they were tense, that her toes had lost their flexibility so that she could not wiggle them, and that the space above the metatarsal arch curved inward instead of being parallel or even curved out. A bunion was beginning to develop, the ankles were swollen and the tissue on the shin-bones was puffy because of the under-functioning of her calf muscles.

This is, unfortunately, a frequent picture of feet and legs in women, and the result is not only headache as a referred pain but many other discomforts, such as sacroiliac trouble and cramps in menstruation.

89

Mrs. Adams was taught how to massage her feet for relaxation, as explained in the following pages; she learned from a simple chart that her body works as a unit and how wrong weight distribution and tense feet with poor circulation brought about her splitting headaches.

By progressive relaxation from the toes to the buttocks, she learned how to use her feet properly, how to improve the functioning of her legs, strengthening the muscles in the calves, thighs and buttocks, with the result that she not only cured her original trouble but greatly improved her posture, her appearance, and her general health. She learned too that she was cured of the cramps that had caused her so much discomfort in starting menstruation.

Foot Troubles

Our poor, abused feet, you see, have a far-reaching effect on our general health, our comfort, and our endurance. Modern people suffer more generally from poor feet than from any other body ailment, as a result of faulty habits and a failure to learn how to use their feet right from earliest childhood. Anyone who has gone through metatarsal trouble knows that these pains in the feet are so agonising that life becomes a burden. Out of a thousand people, the percentage who are completely without foot trouble would be appallingly small.

The most usual sources of trouble are the points marked on the diagram. The over-strained big toe—and in severe cases, bunions—is a result of flabbiness and atrophy at the point marked x. The cause of this over-strain in the big-toe region is wrong weight distribution. Your feet are the key to good posture, to proper alignment, to balance and rhythm of movement. The Chinese have an ancient proverb, "When the big toe is perfect the body is perfect." I go so far as to insist that people with flat feet can seldom be first-class singers or actors, even if they use such artificial means as arch supports to correct their flat feet.

If this seems like an exaggerated statement, experiment for

yourself. Stand with your feet about six inches apart. Carry your weight—where the average person carries his—on the inside of your feet. You will feel a slight sensation of strain in your larynx and around your stomach. It will be difficult to hold your back erect so that your stomach is in. There will be a pull on your inner thighs. Now you begin to understand why lumps form above the knees.

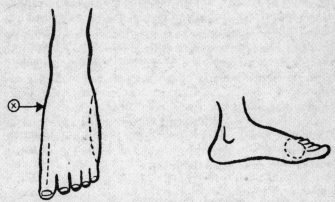

Showing trouble areas on the foot

Flat feet not only are responsible for a great deal of stomach trouble, but they are also frequently a reason for the development of an inferiority complex because they throw the body out of alignment, and only in the poised body is there a poised and balanced personality.

Aching Feet Can Be Cured

It has been my cheering experience that tense and aching feet can be cured at any age. I have had excellent results with pupils as old as sixty-four years. Not long ago, my oldest patient wrote to say, "I bless you every day because I can walk and be active without the slightest discomfort and all the orthopædists whom I had asked for help thought I was too old to improve without special shoes and arch supports."

The feet have infinitely more possibilities for muscular flexibility than the average person dreams. Now and then we encounter the case of people born without arms and discover with astonishment the number of things they learn to do with their feet, keeping them flexible and in excellent working order for a lifetime without aches and pains.

I myself have seen a girl born without arms write by holding a fountain pen between her big toe and second toe, with her writing pad on a low table, some six inches high, resting on the floor. I know of a woman artist in Paris who painted with her feet and was very good at it. Not long ago a national magazine carried pictures of a young woman managing her house-work, cooking, and caring for her baby, all by the intelligent and agile use of her feet.

While most of us are fortunate enough not to have to make such heavy requirements of our feet, we do know that when they are out of working order, we find ourselves suffering from pain, fatigue and related disorders.

Foot-bath for Tense and Aching Feet

This simple foot-bath, if done correctly, will provide an easy and effective treatment for your feet.

Take a chair to the bathroom and place it beside your bath. Sit down and turn on the warm tap to let in enough water to cover your ankles. The water should be agreeably warm; do not let it become too hot. Let your feet hang loose in the water and wiggle your toes once in a while.

Now comes the trick. Every two minutes turn on the hot tap and let a dash of hot water pour in. Repeat eight to ten times, making your foot-bath last twenty minutes. Do not sit in a tense and uncomfortable way, waiting to get through. Sit comfortably relaxed while you read the evening paper or the latest detective story. By pouring in a dash of hot water every two minutes you stimulate blood circulation, which is exactly what we want before you go to bed.

WARNING. Do *not* take this foot-bath when you plan to go out afterwards. It is the following rest that benefits your feet.

The next morning you will be amazed to find how much better your feet feel. In cases of serious foot trouble or great tension, repeat this foot-bath every night for about two weeks; then do it at least three times a week for another two-week period, and once or twice a week until your feet are completely well. You may doubt that such a time will ever come, but I have seen it happen again and again with people who suffered with their feet for years.

If you brush both the tops and soles of your feet with a stiff brush, you will stimulate circulation and arouse nerve sensations.

Treat Your Feet Properly in Summer

In case you suffer in the summer from burning feet and feel exhausted, try this remedy. It feels so good that you will want to make it a habit.

Take off your shoes and stockings and sit on the edge of the bath while you let cold water run over your feet. It will not only relieve your feet but cool your whole body and restore some of the energy you thought you had lost because of the heat. The restoration of vigour to the whole body is well worth the few minutes that this cold bath takes.

What Shoes to Wear

Another hint on being good to your feet before we start our repair work: What about the shoes you wear? During the war, women learned that for any kind of sustained work they had to wear low-heeled shoes on the job. High heels not only endangered their safety in many industrial plants but caused exhaustion. Long hours in high heels will injure the most perfect foot. Too much weight is thrown on the metatarsal arch, which breaks down.

For many years, doctors have issued warnings about the

dangers of high heels. Because of their use, women have three times as many foot defects as men. The satisfaction women derive from this self-inflicted torture in looking taller, in fancy foot gear, is not sufficient compensation for constant pain that affects not only the foot but the welfare of the whole body. Glance around any restaurant or theatre and see women surreptitiously ease their painful, aching feet out of their shoes, and relax with a little sigh of relief. Watch them walk down the street and see the stiff, awkward walk, the cumbersome movements that come as pain increases; the stiffness and strain in their faces; the lack of rhythmical, flowing grace. It is my own belief that any woman who saw herself from the back as she manœuvred herself along the street in high heels, particularly the stilt-like contraptions that have become a recent fashion, would abandon her high heels in horror, except, possibly, for evening wear with long dresses.

It is interesting, by the way, to see pictures of the bone structure of a contemporary woman's foot after some months in one of these stilt shoes and compare it with the deformed foot of one of the old-school Chinese women, whose foot was bound in childhood to keep it small. The effect on the foot is almost exactly the same.

As more and more women become aware of the effect of tension on their health—and on their appearance—the fashion for high heels will probably be left for evening wear, and they will return to the use of shoes that will provide them with comfort and proper support. High heels shorten the Achilles' tendon and prevent proper relaxation, eventually produce wrinkles, make voices sharp, and often are the cause of stomach trouble. Are they worth it?

Low heels, a soft sole and cushioned lining, open toes or heels to provide ventilation give the feet such comfort that one seems to be walking on air. In summer, shoes should be worn one size larger to allow for the swelling that so frequently occurs during the hot months, while white shoes are more healthful in summer because they are many degrees cooler.

94

Releasing Foot Tension

1. Start by shaking your ankles so that your feet move up and down. Your guide for this is the shaking you give your wrist. We are aiming to make your feet move as easily at the ankle as your hands do at the wrist.

Try it. That was a shock, wasn't it? You did not know that your ankles were so stiff. On the day when your ankles are as limber as your wrists, you will have achieved all the relaxation you'll ever want.

2. Massage the feet with a rotating motion. The points marked on the diagram earlier in this chapter are the nerve points where you are apt to find the most trouble.

Particularly give your feet a good rubbing at the inner arch, where you may discover sensitive spots or even real knots. This rubbing may be painful when you first try it and, if so, discontinue the massage for a few days and then try again. But however long it takes, repeat and repeat this foot massage until you can stretch your foot easily and without any feeling of tension or resistance.

Better Weight Distribution

Learn how to stand. Ridiculous, you say. The woman is quite mad. I have been standing all my life.

True, but the chances are that you have not been standing correctly. Perhaps you never learned to stand correctly, even as a small child, for far too often, foot troubles—as you will see in the chapter "How to Prevent Tension in Children"—begin with the first step.

There is only one way to find out how you are standing and distributing your body weight. See for yourself.

Stand in front of a full-length mirror and get acquainted with the functioning of those feet of yours. Perhaps you belong to the "toes out" school. It is almost incredible what this misunderstood foot position has done to several generations.

Place your feet straight so that big toe and heel form one straight line.

After you have checked your position in the mirror, to make sure that your feet are straight, close your eyes to help you get the sensation of proper weight distribution.

When you stand with the toes turned out, you weaken your lower back. When the feet are straight your knees are strong and you have more strength in hips and lower back. Standing with toes out weakens the buttocks. Straight feet give you strong buttocks.

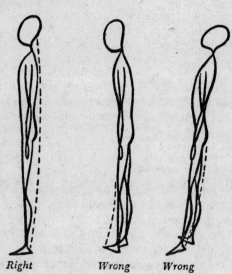

Right   Wrong   Wrong

Showing the right way to stand for proper weight distribution and two positions you should avoid

You will realise how important the position of your feet is when you stop to think of the bearing that it has upon your whole upright position, your sense of alignment and balance. Proper use of the feet is as vital for you as the proper foundations for a building.

Another feature of standing with the feet straight is that it enables the toes to move flexibly. With the toes out you cannot do this because you overload your inner arch and block your big toe. Also the sole of the foot becomes more flexible so that you can curl it up.

Now take another look in the mirror. This time examine the position of your ankles. If they sag to the inside, pull them up about half an inch until they are erect, and once more close your eyes until you know how this position feels. Instead of the weight being on the inside of your legs, pulling down, the weight coming from your hip goes over your knees, and puts to work the outside of feet and arches.

As a result, the inner arch is relieved of weight; the lazy muscle group around the ankles gets to work and the small bones that were out of place in your so-called flat feet gradually slip back into position.

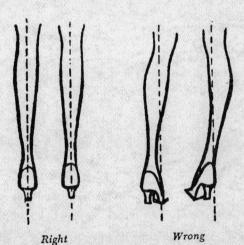

Right   Wrong

Showing the position of the feet for proper weight distribution, and a position to avoid

Proper weight distribution and right function, in other

words, will correct your flat feet and give you a new sensation of power and confidence as you improve your weight distribution.

The Leg Stretch

In learning this stretch, you must be careful to do it correctly. Properly performed, it is one of the most beneficial of habits. Wrongly done, it creates more tension and worse feet.

Lie comfortably on your bed or couch and close your eyes. By closing your eyes, you can shut out all distractions and concentrate on your sensations.

Now begin to stretch your leg. The initiative for the movement must start above your heel at the Achilles' tendon and *not with the muscles of the foot*.

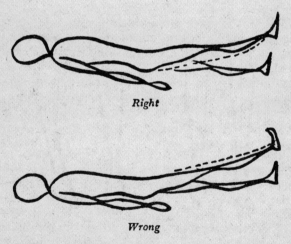

Right

Wrong

Showing right and wrong ways of doing the leg stretch, and where you feel the pull

Push the heel forward as though you were trying to push a wall away. If you do this properly you will feel the stretching sensation up through your calf to the knee and—if no nerve sensation is blocked by tension—up your thigh to the small of your back.

The difficulty is that the foot muscles move more quickly than the muscles above the heel, and the foot will lift itself up before you can start pushing the heel. When you feel your foot pulling up, relax and start over again. And again. And again. Until you feel that the stretch is starting where it should, in the back. The foot will become so relaxed that it will follow the initiative of the heel instead of taking the lead.

If the ankles feel very stiff when you start, try shaking them as you shake your wrists to relax your hands. This movement is worth any effort because when you have once mastered it, you will prevent your feet from getting stiff and overloaded, keep your calves in proper function—and the proper shape— your thighs in working condition, and help to strengthen your lower back muscles and keep them fit.

When you feel that you are doing it properly, alternate, doing first one leg, then the other. Once you can do it lying down, try it standing up and you will feel the pull clear to your shoulder-blades.

Try this leg stretch now and then when you are sitting at work and you will be surprised how much more alive your whole body will feel.

Relief for Tired Toes

When you have developed a sensation in the region of the Achilles' tendon that goes down to your heels and makes you use them for proper standing and walking, you will be able to relieve your toes of weight-carrying. The toes were not meant to carry weight. Their function—in our primitive, barefoot ancestors—was to sense the ground before the foot rested on it. The weight should be so distributed that the toes are free. What happens? Well, the metatarsal arches become stronger and more flexible, you can move your toes freely, thus stimulating circulation. And, most important of all, your

99

feet, once flexible and free of weight, will become a main source of relaxation instead of a main source of pain, tension, and fatigue.

Treatment for Bunions

Bunions develop when the big toe muscles and ligaments are over-strained, and in many cases the last joint of the big toe is additionally exposed to pressure from a shoe that is either too short or too narrow. If you have a bunion, try the following treatment:

1. Make the foot-bath a daily habit.
2. Massage the big toe, starting at the point A on the diagram, between the big toe and the second toe.

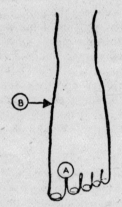

Points to massage on the foot

3. Massage the point marked B at the inner arch.
4. Rotate the big toe to give it increased flexibility.
5. Practise rising on your tiptoes, so that you feel the pull on your arch. Take hold of a chair back to balance yourself. Rise on the tips of your toes, lower the foot slightly but not

enough so that the heel will touch the ground. Now up and down several times.

As soon as the normal position of the big toe is regained, and space established between the other toes, the inflammation that caused the pain in the bunion will disappear.

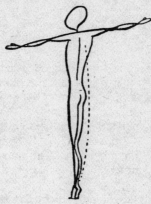

Showing correct position for rising on tiptoes without support

Many people who had been under the care of chiropodists for years have told me that their chiropodists were amazed at the improvement in their feet after several weeks' practise of this technique.

CHAPTER EIGHT

The Release of Tense Leg Muscles

I AM sure you belong to the millions who, because of uncomfortable chairs, have acquired the habit of sitting for hours with crossed legs.

Sitting with crossed legs is a damaging habit. "But why," you protest, "when it is so much more comfortable?"

Well, let's see what it really does to your body.

1. It is bad for your lower back because it pulls your spine out of shape.

2. Instead of sitting on the parts of your thighs that were designed for that purpose, you develop a habit of sitting on spread buttocks.

3. Crossed legs prevent proper circulation of blood to the internal organs and prevent them from functioning properly.

4. Crossed legs make the thigh muscles tense, press on the knees, and are one reason for the ugly lumps that form on the inner side of the knees, which we will try to correct later.

In case you have acquired this habit, be very strict with yourself. Each time you find yourself in this position, uncross your legs. At first you will find this annoying and believe that you are less comfortable, but once you get accustomed to sitting properly you will realise that it makes you feel better.

Try, if you can, to find a chair that lets you put your feet on the floor, and then keep them there. It is all right, by the way, to cross your ankles.

Sit properly in front of a mirror and notice the difference. With the lower back straight instead of curved, you will feel more relaxed from the waist up as the pressure on your abdomen is released.

One of the most frequent complaints of drivers of motor-cars, vans and taxicabs is of pain in the right leg and knee. Frequently, the sufferer believes that he has developed either rheumatism or arthritis. Heat treatments are started which give relief for a while but in time the pain starts again. The person who fears he has arthritis or rheumatism tries not to use the painful knee in order to "spare" it; and at the same time he develops a psychological complex because he associates these complaints with age, and subconsciously he begins to act as if he were old.

Let us look at the driver's knee from the point of view of function. The driver, like the average user of a sewing machine or piano, keeps his knee stretched, creating a pull as shown in the drawing, and each down movement produces a strain on the muscles behind the knee. In time, the muscles

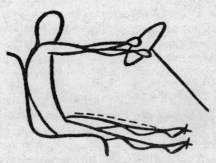

The wrong way to sit when you drive. The broken line shows where the leg feels strain

revolt and begin to hurt in order to call attention to their misuse. The driver, who if his motor developed trouble would get at the source of it, is less kind to his own body. He simply tries to stop the pain without attempting to understand the cause.

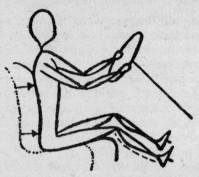

How you should sit when you drive. Dotted line indicates outline of the seat before adjustment. Broken line shows where you should feel the pull.

The pain is a result of an improper position at the wheel which throws strain on the ankle, leg and knee muscles. Adjust the seat so that you can reach the pedal with the knee bent instead of stretched, or fit a pillow behind your back to bring you forward and relieve the tension.

After a short time, the proper use of your leg will restore not only flexibility but also strength to the weak muscles.

Tension After Operations

Many people come to me with stiff arms and legs which are a product of tension after an operation as a result of which the limb had to be kept more or less immobile for some time. Without realising that the source of the trouble is simply lack of use, these people believe that the leg or arm is actually unable to function.

One such case was that of a young woman who, some years before, had suffered from an accident while ski-ing. She had developed a weakness in her right knee and she had tried the usual remedies, heat treatments and massage, without relief. As her fiancé enjoyed athletic sports, she was most unhappy because she believed she would never be able to share them with him.

What actually had happened was that the nerve sensations in this leg had become blocked above the knee and never restored, so she had developed an awkward walk that made her feel insecure, which added to the awkwardness. I taught her how to massage the leg and immediately after each treatment made her use the re-established sensation to restore muscle function. It took us only six weeks to restore flexibility to the leg and she once more became a skilful skier.

A fifteen-year-old boy was brought to my office. For five years he had been in a hospital. He had had an injury for which several operations were performed and the leg was kept in a cast. By the end of five years it was completely stiff. That meant no sports, no games for ever. And he was a normal fifteen-year-old boy, who for five years had lived in a hospital with no outlet for his energies, no real companionship with other boys.

"And yet," he told me wistfully, "there was nothing wrong with me. It was only my leg."

Could I do something for him? Well, after examining the leg, I did not believe that it was really stiff; I suspected that it was only very tense. I started to relieve this tension around the knee at all the nerve centres I could reach with my fingers. And the miracle that was no miracle happened. The knee began to move again.

As it happened, this boy's difficulties were increased because he had been released without orthopædic shoes. In the beginning of our treatments one leg was an inch shorter than the other; every time he used the right leg he lurched forward. We had a simple lift made by a shoemaker which relieved this difficulty in walking, enabled him to develop his trunk properly, and eased up the amount of effort which each step cost him. At the end of five weeks he came to me, as happy as a boy can be, because he was able to play baseball. He has kept up his sports ever since, earns his living, and is able to bend his knee forty-five degrees.

His was one of many orthopædic cases in which so much tension had settled in a muscle group that it appeared to be permanently stiff. Since Bill uses his leg constantly, bending it as he runs and walks up and down stairs, he needs no further treatments. He is improving in the natural way, through use.

A woman came to my office in Florence, Italy, seeking help because she felt insecure in walking and often fell, for no understandable reason. She was planning to live with her daughter in the Swiss Alps and, because of her sense of insecurity, she dreaded the winters with snow and icy roads. Could I help her strengthen her feet?

When I tried to trace the cause of her disturbed balance, I discovered that not only her left arm was so weak that she could not perform swinging or lifting movements; but her left leg, knee and the back muscles on the left side were nearly atrophied.

"What happened to you?" I asked.

Ten years before, she explained, she had broken her left arm. It was a simple break but while the arm was in a cast she had developed an awkward walk. Because she could not swing her left arm freely, she overloaded the right side, hip and leg.

After the arm was removed from the cast, she continued to move cautiously until she had made a habit of wrong body alignment. Hence the frequent falls and her feeling of insecurity. By re-establishing a proper sense of body alignment and releasing the tense muscle groups and developing those that had fallen into disuse, she recovered so completely that she wrote me jubilantly that she had gone through the whole severe winter without a single fall.

This lack of re-education after accidents or operations results in countless cases of improper muscular function.

Breathing

What does breathing have to do with the proper function of your legs? Well, when you get the tank of your car filled with

106

petrol, you ask the garage man to check the air in your tyres. You know that you must have exactly the right pressure if the tyres are to last and the car is to run smoothly.

Your legs, knees, and feet serve as your tyres. If your breathing is shallow, the muscles of your sides and back do not expand. That means that the air pressure is not evenly distributed and some parts of the body machine are overloaded; the inner side of the legs, for instance, bringing bumps around the knees and trouble to the tense big toe.

Two thousand years before Christ, the Chinese had a proverb that declared, "The healthy man breathes with his big toe; the sick man with his throat."

Your Thighs

There is another source of disturbance that is often overlooked, and that is the thighs. Here again that habit of improper sitting takes its toll; it is responsible for enlarging the thigh as well as the hip.

Both men and women discover with considerable surprise the cost of neglecting the proper function of the thighs.

In women, this awareness generally comes at the beginning of the bathing season when they try on a bathing suit before a mirror and discover with horror that they have accumulated flabby tissue above the knees which is much too unsightly to make a good appearance on the beach.

It is a different story with men who are apt to have developed tension in the thighs through being muscle-bound. How often men have come to me, complaining about nervous tension, insomnia, and frequently sex difficulties. In these cases, I often find that they are muscle-bound.

"Did you play baseball when at school?" I asked.

"Yes," they acknowledge in surprise, obviously wondering what baseball has to do with their insomnia and their other difficulties.

I point out then, what I have reiterated so often in this book, that muscle activity must be balanced. If one group is overloaded and another is under-worked, there is no proper balance. In these cases, the muscles of the thighs were developed by baseball far more than the trunk muscles, and as a result they were now unable to release tension. Before they could get rid of their troubles, they had to learn to relax these thigh muscles and develop adequate trunk muscles.

In most cases, this suggestion is bitterly resented. Frequently enough, these thigh muscles are the only really developed muscles they have and they are very proud of them.

How to Relax Tense Thigh Muscles

The best way to relax tense thigh muscles is to massage the points of nerve centres under and at both sides of the knee.

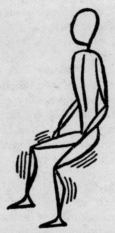

How to shake the knees and thighs for relaxing tense thigh muscles

After giving them a good rubbing and kneading, sit on a chair with your feet six inches apart, and start to shake your thighs and knees from side to side, in the same way that you flapped your hands up and down at the wrist. You are aiming for the same sensation of looseness. The more loosely relaxed you sit, the more you will be aware of a tingling sensation all through the thighs, knees, calves, down to your toes.

When you have mastered this thigh relaxation, pull up your lower back and you will be able to sit on the proper part of your thighs.

In cases where the front muscles of the thighs are tense and the back muscles are flabby, try the leg stretch (see page 98) when you have finished the shaking and you will be able to develop a proper balance in the use of these muscles.

The Knee Drop

Another method of relieving tension in the thighs is the knee drop.

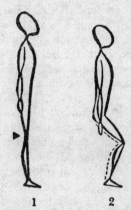

1   2

Steps in doing the knee drop. Arrowhead shows where to begin the movement, broken line indicates where you feel the sensation.

Stand with your feet six inches apart and parallel, then let your knees get so weak that they sink down, as though they were giving way under you. Close your eyes while you do it so that you can be more strongly aware of the sensation it gives you. Repeat several times and observe how relaxed your thigh muscles become.

How to Correct Flabby Thighs

A great many women are afflicted with flabby thighs. Stand in front of the mirror and find out whether you are the possessor of the so-called bumps above your knees.

These bumps are a result of faulty weight distribution that overloads the inner arch of your foot and puts a strain on it, as well as overtaxes the big toe. In many cases, people who suffer from these bumps above the knees also suffer from metatarsal pains. The misshapen thighs, in other words, have the root of their trouble in the wrong use of your feet.

How do we start to correct this unattractive condition?

1. First, develop proper habits of breathing, without which you cannot acquire the proper posture.

2. Sit on a chair with feet loosely resting on the floor, and begin a short rotating rubbing, first directly on the bumps, and then in the whole area of the bumps. Don't be alarmed if it hurts in the beginning. Wait for a few days and then begin again.

3. When you start to feel a sensation of aliveness in this flabby tissue as a result of stimulation of the nerves, begin the leg stretch (see page 98). Make sure that you start the stretch not with the foot but at the Achilles' tendon. Stretch so that you can feel a pulling sensation from the outside of the ankle, up the outside of the leg to the hip. As soon as you feel the stretch at the outside and not on the inside, you know you are beginning to revive the activity of these sluggish muscles which have not participated in walking and standing as much as they should.

Keep at it for some weeks and your bumps will be gone, your walk will improve, and your feet will be grateful to you for having relieved them of the strain they must carry when overloaded.

4. The knee drop (see page 109) is beneficial for this condition.

5. Walking up and down stairs is also useful to people with flabby thighs. Once you learn proper alignment of the body, and remember to use your breath to help you in climbing, you will find that the nervous palpitations which frighten so many people will disappear. Functional movement is performed without effort, and it is a pleasure to do it. When a movement is an effort, you are performing it improperly. It is wise to remember that instead of saying, "It tires me," you should say, "I am tiring myself. This is absurd. Why should I be so hard on myself? Let's take it easy."

Relaxing the Legs

As I have pointed out before, the time to relax is not after you are tired, but while you are in the process of becoming tired, or—ideally—before you get tired.

Here are some methods of relaxing the legs:

1. Stretch the legs several times and make the stretch a habit. (Obviously, not while the boss is standing beside your desk.)

2. Remember that the tensest spot is apt to be the ankles. Shake them up and down. Keep it up. No one is going to notice your feet flying about under your desk. When those ankles become really flexible, you will bless me for the feeling of relaxation you get.

3. If you have flabby knees, with sagging knee caps, rub around those flabby bumps until you feel that some sensation has been aroused. (NOTE: Unless you arouse a nerve sensation first, the movements in themselves will not be of much benefit to you. Precede the movements by the massaging.)

4. Now do the leg stretch (page 98). When you have done that, stand with your feet six inches apart and pull the knee cap of one leg in, making the pull so strong that you feel the muscles in the back of the knee pulling like a rope. Let the knee cap relax, and repeat.

In the beginning, you may feel a lot of resistance, but keep it up. Make it a daily habit, doing it dozens of times a day, while waiting for a bus, standing in queues, and so forth. When you have mastered it, you can do it so inconspicuously that no one will notice.

These knee cap pulls and ankle relaxers are a godsend to people who spend a great deal of time standing, such as waiters, shop assistants, beauty parlour operators, and others, as they relieve fatigue and pain in legs and feet.

CHAPTER NINE

The Back, Your Body's Stepchild

THE back is the stepchild of the modern human body. Stand before a full-length mirror, undressed, and, with a hand mirror, look at yourself from the back. Take your time. Study your posture, the position of your shoulders, the alignment of your spine, your buttocks. How many of the vital muscle groups in your back are tense from overwork? How many of them are flabby because you aren't making the proper use of them?

You see now why I said at the outset that there is little point to harping on posture until the muscles are in shape to carry out their proper functions.

What has gone wrong to get your back in that condition, or was it ever properly developed in childhood? Major accidents? Probably just the little things, the wrong use that has become a habit. Our old enemy, the sixteen-hour sitting position, for one thing. For instance, wrong sitting habits have a lot to do with those flabby buttocks which cause not only unsightly appearance but creates more trouble than the average man or woman ever realises.

How to Strengthen Flabby Buttocks

Flabby buttocks have the same effect on the body that a flat tyre has on your car; your whole body is wrongly aligned. Not only are your inner organs affected by the functioning of your buttocks but also the back of your neck and head suffer from tension as a result of this unbalanced position of the muscles of the back.

Try it for yourself. Sit on a chair and see what your flabby buttocks do to your lower back. Your spine curves out. Now pull up your lower back and sit on your upper thighs so that you feel a pull in the sides and the lower part of the thighs.

What happens? You not only look much taller but you discover that your shoulder-blades feel relaxed and your neck is straighter. Your head loses its down pull.

Instead of feeling heavy, you feel pounds lighter and, when you turn, you no longer feel cumbersome but have a sensation of pivoting around.

Men and women should be aware of the importance of preventing or eliminating this flabbiness in the buttocks and of the necessity of sitting properly. In the chapter on "Sex and Common Sense" I will explain why this is of such far-reaching importance and what the elimination of flabby thighs can do in the process of rejuvenation.

How are you to correct those flabby buttocks aside from learning to sit properly?

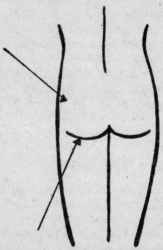

To correct flabby buttocks, pull in and up at the points indicated

Well, look at the accompanying diagram, and pull the buttocks up and in at the points indicated. Do this not once or twice a day but dozens of times. Keep at it, over and over, whenever you think of it. You will not be able to correct this flabbiness in a day or a week. It will take many weeks. But it will be worth it. In time the muscles will become so strong that it will be instinctive to sit on the right spot. Once you acquire proper function, you won't need to keep up the pulling movement. The proper habit will be all that is necessary to keep them in condition. But at the start you must pull and pull until you have regained the firm, small shape that they should have.

Too many women think that they can achieve the same effect by wearing a rubber girdle that presses the buttocks together so that they do not look flabby. The rubber girdle, however, has no effect on the flabby tissue and muscles, nor does it help to tone up the muscles of the whole system. It merely deceives the eye of the observer. Make no mistake about it, firm buttock muscles not only make you move like a younger person but they make you feel younger. I have yet to see a girdle that can accomplish that.

There is no age limit for this improving of the buttocks. Men and women of sixty and over were able to strengthen these muscles, improve their internal organs and their blood and lymph circulation, and get rid of that feeling of weight around the abdominal cavity.

Developing the Buttocks

1. Practise the leg stretch (see page 98) to wake up this dead area.
2. A constant pulling in and up of the buttocks will be helpful. You can do this while you are waiting for the bus or as a strap-hanger on your way to work.
3. Use the proper sitting position (see page 113). And here again let me remind you not to cross your legs, which throws the body completely out of alignment.
4. Do plenty of walking. Walk with a swing from the small of your back. This walk, as contrasted to walking from the

top of the thighs, means all the difference between effort and pleasure. Why make the necessary activities of everyday life difficult for yourself when they can add up to so much enjoyment?

The person who is physically at the peak of his vitality is a happy person. He carries a glow around with him. The perfect well-being of the body creates a zest for living that is sheer delight. This is the baby's zest. It is a zest that is your right. The extent to which you fall short of it—and only the smallest fraction of us do not fall short of it—is the gauge of the improper functioning of your body. And nine times out of ten, it is simply because you are trying too hard, and consequently doing things the wrong way.

The swinging walk not only refreshes you, but it restores your personal breathing rhythm. And remember that when your breathing rhythm is undisturbed, you are most yourself; your personality is flowering.

As our cities become more crowded, the simple exercise of walking becomes more and more of a problem. I agree that it is difficult to walk with the right swing in crowded streets, because your natural pace must be altered to allow for the people jostling you on either side, and you have to weave in and out.

Most of us are such creatures of habit that we automatically walk along the same streets, without regard to our own comfort. If the street on which you usually walk is exceptionally crowded, think for a minute. Perhaps there is another street with fewer pedestrians. Suppose it is a little out of your way? It is worth the extra few steps to be able to walk with full enjoyment.

Your Lower Back

Study the muscles of the lower back. It will very likely come as a surprise to realise how strong this part of the body should be if all the muscles were really functioning properly.

And yet the lower back tends to be neglected and to grow weak because of—yes, you guessed it!—our sitting habits and the fact that contemporary sedentary life offers little real work for these muscles to do.

Those long muscles of the back, which hold the vertebræ in place, extend from the back of the skull to the pelvis, at either side of the spine. They are fortified by many other muscle groups, particularly in the region of the small of the back.

Elderly People—Lower Back

My experience has shown that all age groups respond to the change that comes with the strengthening of the lower back and buttocks.

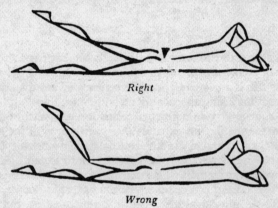

Right

Wrong

To do the leg lift properly, pull up leg, starting at the small of the back (shown by arrowhead). Do not bend the leg.

A well-known college professor came to me for help in relieving an ache in the lower back that had troubled him for about twenty years. He was so uncomfortable when he sat down that he had acquired an awkward and distorted position to help relieve the pain.

117

The reason for the weakness in the small of the back was an accident of many years past that had not been followed by re-education in muscular habits. It took terrific strength, and kneading with my knuckles, before I could restore any sensation in the atrophied muscles of that region. As soon as some feeling was restored, we started to develop the muscles.

The best method to develop muscles in this part of the back is by lying comfortably, face down, on a bed or couch that supports the whole body; then pull up the legs, starting at the small of the back.

After three months of working on this muscle re-education, he was able to begin to swim in the sea, which he had abandoned years before, and the breast stroke helped to restore the muscles of the lower back. As proper function was re-established, the pain disappeared.

Back Breathing While Sitting

Another habit to strengthen your lower back is to use the small of your back for expansion while you breathe. For most people this is a completely new experience. They live with the idea that breathing affects only their chest.

Of course, you do not actually breathe in your lower back, but as the diaphragm expands downwards and all the organs below the diaphragm are involved in its movements, you can see that your lower back actually is able to expand far more than you ever realised. This expansion, that takes place each time you inhale, especially when you are sitting down, keeps the whole muscle group of the lower back in condition, because the muscles take part in each expansion, keeping them flexible, preventing atrophy. Learning to breathe so that these muscles take part in the action has cured innumerable cases of lower back pain.

Experiment for yourself and see how these muscles work. Sit on a chair and put both hands on your hips, thumbs forward so that the fingers are turned to the back. First practise a long, deep yawn. When you have done that, and are aware of the feeling of expansion in your muscles, breathe deeply, so that the diaphragm expands and the muscles take part in the movement. When you have learned to make that a habit, you will not need to think of it and the flexibility of the muscles will strengthen your lower back.

The Back Bend

This is one of the most important techniques in the whole book. Stand with your feet several inches apart, knees straight. The head starts the movement by loosening up completely in the neck and pulling down the spine gradually through its weight of about eight pounds. The farther the head drops the more vertebræ are involved. Finally you will feel the bend all the way to your rectum. As you bend, exhale slowly.

When you have bent as far as you can go, swing back and forth from the hips, and then start to breathe in the lower back between ribs and pelvis.

Hold your breath, and while you feel the breath act as a support for the upward movement, begin to pull the muscles above the buttocks. That is the point at which your up-swing should start. Gradually pull yourself up, so that you have the sensation of imitating a cat by rolling up one vertebra after another until your back is straight. Your head is still bent and you are still full of air. Now gradually pull your shoulder-blades together, and your head will follow so that you stand erect.

When you have mastered this back bend it will remain your best relaxation habit and refresher whenever you have to be at your best and have no time in which to take a nap. It will bring the blood back into your head and take the stiffness out of your back, and give you the feeling of waking from a restful sleep.

Many bankers and executives have told me that they practise this bending before strenuous meetings, with excellent results. It is also invaluable to artists, singers, actors and dancers before going on the stage.

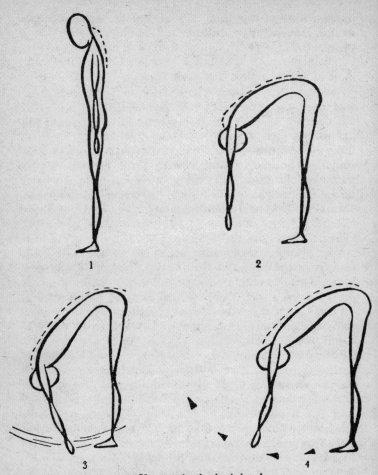

How to do the back bend

In the beginning you will have trouble when you start to come up after the bend, because the usual method is to push up below the shoulder-blades. This is of no use to us, however, as our purpose is to strengthen those poorly functioning muscles of the lower back. Be patient in keeping at this because it pays.

Stomach In

And now that we have checked the muscle groups from head to toe, and know which ones need overhauling, we realise that once we establish the proper function, our posture will take care of itself.

But look here, you protest indignantly, you haven't said a word about the most important thing of all, the thing all the beauty editors tell us, and the gymnasium instructors, and the authorities who tell us how to be young, beautiful and graceful in one easy lesson. You haven't said anything about "Keep your stomach in".

Well, the proof of the pudding is in the eating. Stand up and pull your stomach in, according to the popular rules. Now try to take a good deep breath. You can't? Of course you can't. What's happening inside while you pull your stomach in? That pull of external muscles is blocking the diaphragm and preventing its downward expansion. When the diaphragm can't expand downward, the lower organs fail to get the kind of stimulation they need.

Every time you pull your stomach in, you are creating an unreleased tension. This habit is responsible for pain and cramps in menstruation, and for constipation; it can cause gall-bladder and stomach trouble. It can cause unreleased fears and heart conditions. And the irony of the whole stomach-in position is that the pull weakens your back and in the long run makes your posture worse.

What then? Well, instead of going to all the effort of pulling in and creating tensions, suppose you take it easy and do it the natural way.

Stand at ease and let your abdomen relax. Now inhale deeply and exhale with a sharp shhing sound by pursing your lips, imitating a child playing choo-choo.

Now what happened? Your abdominal muscles automatically pulled in strongly, not only in the middle but far to the sides. And the shh that accompanied the exhalation affected your internal breathing muscles, causing a sensation of stimulation through the whole body and a deep and natural demand for another long breath.

Now pull your stomach in again and observe that the feeling of tension extends clear up to your larynx. The lower part of your lungs is prevented from filling with air. The diaphragm can't perform its soft down movement. You are depriving your blood of oxygen.

Worst of all, when you pull your stomach in, you block the flexibility of your ribs, which is of immense importance for the action of your heart. The greater the flexibility of the chest cavity, the easier it is for the heart to expand and pump. When you stop to consider the increase in heart conditions to-day, surely it is only commonsense to give the heart a break. Make the work of your organs as easy as you can for yourself.

Improved Appetite

Over and over again I have observed the improvement in appetite that comes to people who work with me for the correction of weak backs or curvature of the spine.

There was a young woman of thirty who suffered from curvature of the spine and who, in spite of expert orthopædic care, was tense and had many atrophied muscles. She had tried in vain to increase her weight. Even insulin treatments and hospitalisation had been tried without result. She was still under-weight and had a poor appetite when she came to me.

My first task in her case was to bring flexibility to her spine in the region of the thoracic vertebræ and to improve her breathing. As soon as she learned how to loosen up her chest and to relax around the abdomen, she began to enjoy eating and to discover that she could eat many dishes that had, in the past, been too difficult for her to digest. Lack of appetite had been a result of the tension caused by the curvature of the spine and, as that was the case, none of the treatments had helped until the tension was released.

And this brings me to a point that is of vital importance in the rebuilding of muscle groups. That is the matter of proper diet. It is essential that your diet contain the proper vitamins if you are to show the best results. If you are not sure what foods and in what quantities you should have for your own personal needs, consult your physician. Don't guess at it.

CHAPTER TEN

How to Stay Well and Live Longer

MODERN science has come to realise that tension is an underlying cause not only in mental illness, but in physical illness as well. Its effect on the organs is of great importance. By learning how to achieve a correct release of tension, it is possible to attack illness at the right point—at the very beginning—and so to prevent the organs from being thrown out of order. It is a better thing to stay well than to get well.

So far we have learned how to correct muscular tension by training the muscles for proper function, and acquiring the proper alignment of the body on these well-functioning muscles, the body and movements supported always by correct breathing.

Now let's see what tension can do to the organs of the body.

The Heart and Tension

It is becoming increasingly apparent that a tremendous number of people who believe that they have heart trouble are suffering entirely from nervous tension. They exhibit many of the same symptoms, the racing heart and the palpitations, shortness of breath and dizziness, pain around the heart and sometimes even unconsciousness.

After examination, however, the perplexed doctor finds that the heart itself is not diseased. What then is disturbing its function? The trouble lies in nervous tensions of which the heart ailment is merely a symptom. And the nervous tensions, frequently enough, grow out of an initial condition of impaired breathing.

In many cases, the root of the difficulty is a stiffness in the intercostals, the muscles between the ribs, which, in deep breathing, expand with each inhalation and thus are kept flexible. When the breathing is shallow and impaired, the muscles are not called upon to do enough work and they grow stiff. It is a curious thing—and we will discuss it later—that a tight muscle at this point creates a fear complex. No one can completely release a sensation of physical fear while there is tension in this muscle. And the fear complex inevitably leads to more tension, to a racing heart, to more impaired breathing.

I recall a woman of forty-five who came to me, complaining of heart trouble. Doctors had told her that there was no organic trouble. I found that the intercostals above the heart were as tense as steel. When she was able to relieve her tension and breathe deeply, the condition cleared up.

Not only so-called nervous heart conditions are due to un-released tension, but also the ailments associated with a high-standing diaphragm. For instance, false angina pectoris, that occurs when the diaphragm stands too high because of gas formation, belongs to this category. Because of the pain, this is a frightening ailment and one that is easily relieved.

Relaxation and Heart Trouble

On the other hand, people with real heart trouble can obtain considerable relief through relaxation and improved breathing which relieves the strain on the chest.

After an attack of angina pectoris, the president of a great foundation was referred to me by his doctor. Relaxation through breathing, the doctor said, would be most beneficial. I found the patient's chest around the heart very tense and the intercostals rigid.

A real heart condition is not, obviously, a case for violent measures, so we started carefully and gradually to restore proper breathing habits, progressing slowly so as to avoid any additional strain on the heart. When the chest muscles began to relax, he felt great relief and we then took up light physical exercises. But it was not enough in his case—*or in any case*—simply to restore muscular flexibility. Unless this changed habit becomes a part of daily living, it serves no real function. The purpose of this book is not merely to show you how to use your body, but how to use it for greater joy in living.

Planning the Day

Along with the relaxation habits, therefore, we worked out a new plan for living so that the patient could get through his day's work with less strain; there was no attempt to curtail the amount of work he did; he knew best what had to be accomplished. My job was to show him how to do his work and, at the same time, to take it easy.

First, a couch was placed in his office. Thirty minutes before lunch, his secretary saw to it that no one entered his office and that no telephone call was put through. All morning he had the assurance that at twelve-thirty he would have a completely undisturbed rest period in which to lie on his couch. Sometimes he took a nap, sometimes he read, at other times he simply lay as quietly as he could, watching his body relax. But, under all circumstances, he spent his half-hour in complete privacy.

The result was not only physical, it was psychological as well. It meant that even when he had to see a great many people and had a rushed morning schedule, he was free of the fear—"This will be too much for me." He knew that there was a period for rest and recuperation ahead.

The second change was in the direction of simplifying his life. He had been using his lunch-time—like an overwhelming number of business men—as a time for business conferences. Meal-times should always be a period of rest. When it is accompanied by strain, tension develops, and frequently stomach complaints.

We planned that henceforth he would make only two lunch engagements a week and the rest of the time he would eat alone in some quiet place where he would be neither hurried nor disturbed.

I was able to follow up his case for several years. At the end of that time he felt well, had lost his fear of having a recurrence of his attacks, and he was grateful that he had learned how to use his strength intelligently and to keep his budget of energy balanced.

The Sensitive Stomach

Recent cancer research has revealed that in many cases of gastric cancer—cancer of the stomach—the patient has far too little digestive fluid in his stomach. Frequently, this failure to produce enough digestive fluid is due to shallow breathing and consequent tension around the middle of the trunk.

In other cases, the tension is caused by the conditions under which meals are eaten. The hurry, noise, and strain of a busy cafeteria, for instance, can play havoc with the digestive processes.

It is the part of wisdom for every individual to examine his daily habits, to ask himself: "Does this condition give me a sense of strain? Do I relax better under such-and-such circumstances?" The causes are manifold, but in all cases it is your own recognition of your tension and your knowledge of how to release it that brings about improvement.

The stomach is sensitive and immediately responsive to nerve tension. The phrase "He makes me sick" has an element of truth. The thing that upsets you, the person who irritates you, the van that just missed you in traffic and frightened you, all these things have a reaction on the stomach. They make you sick.

How Mental Attitudes Influence the Stomach

A young man came to me for relief from stomach trouble.

127

Investigation had revealed that he did not have enough digestive fluid in his stomach.

I asked what was worrying him. He was aware that he was too highly strung and he tried to describe his mental condition to me.

"I live," he said, "under a constant drive of being rushed. Wherever I am, I feel that I should be somewhere else. Whatever I do, I am tormented by the thought that I should be doing the next thing. I constantly have the feeling that I am missing something, as though something were always escaping me. I grope for it but I can't reach it because I can never bring my full mind to bear on it. My conscious mind is always rushing ahead of my body. My mind and my body don't seem to be in the same place at the same time."

I explained to him that he shared this feeling with many, many other people. Particularly those who are especially gifted and ambitious seem to be unable to release the tension that produces this state of mind.

We started relaxation and breathing techniques, and it was interesting to observe how, as he learned to release tension, he learned to live fully in the moment, mentally and physically. At the end of a few months his stomach trouble had disappeared.

Tension and Ulcers

Just as tension may be responsible for too little digestive fluid, so it can be responsible for too much fluid, which is an attendant condition with stomach ulcers.

It is, however, not enough to know that tension may cause the ulcers. The main point is to find out *what habit causes the tension and how it can be eliminated.*

A woman pianist came to my office after having suffered for many years from stomach and duodenal ulcers. Recently, she said, the ulcers had grown worse rather than better, although she followed the strictest sort of diet.

In the course of describing her ailment, the kind of treatments she had had, and the rest of her medical history, she told me a great deal about herself and her life.

She told me that she had been educated by a strict mother, whose training limited the child's movements to the small field of what she considered lady-like. She never really played with abandon, or gave her muscles the sort of work-out that they should have had. She never found her own personal rhythm but from early childhood was hedged in by taboos which resulted in restricted movement. To add to this, her mother's constant admonition was, "Be careful! Don't run. Don't strain yourself. Your father has heart trouble and you may have inherited it."

The result of this training was a constant holding back of natural movements and attendant tension. But, while the child was not allowed to play naturally, she was forced to sit for long hours practising on the piano, after coming home from school. And yet she did not understand why she had stomach ulcers!

To her surprise I waved her towards my grand piano. "Sit down and play for me," I said.

She did so and I watched her carefully. I observed that she was extremely tense through her abdomen while she played, that her breathing was shallow and that she pressed on her stomach without releasing this pressure when she exhaled.

I explained to her what her wrong habit was and what she could do to correct the situation.

First I taught her to relax while lying down. When she could do this properly, and when she had learned how to yawn so deeply that her whole abdomen relaxed, I had her sit at the piano.

"Play," I said, "but watch yourself. Be aware of your own sensations. Find out how you are using your body."

She began to play and in a little while broke off and nodded her head. She was amazed by the tension that began almost at once in the region of the stomach. (NOTE: This is why I constantly stress the awakening of sensations. For the most part, people are not aware of their own tensions and of their own bad habits. Only when the sensations are aroused, are they conscious of how their bodies function.)

"What can I do about it?" she asked.

First, Track Down the Bad Habit

The first step, I pointed out, was to be aware of the habit. The next and obvious step was to correct the habit. She knew now that her breathing and her tension around the stomach were causing the trouble. She must watch her new way of breathing until it functioned automatically. She must be aware of the stomach tension. As soon as she became aware of it, she was to stop practising and lie down for a few minutes until she had become completely relaxed before she resumed her playing.

Her trouble was a bad habit of many years' standing and it takes will power and patience to overcome such a habit. When, however, the sufferer knows that the habit brings with it constant and increasing pain, there is a steady reminder to help in keeping at the cure. With patience, then, this woman got rid of her ulcers and had no recurrence.

But while cancer and ulcers are serious problems, an infinite amount of misery, discomfort, poor health, and gloom follow such results of tension as indigestion and constipation. The amount of money spent on laxatives, digestive remedies and patent medicines is appalling. None of it gets at the root of the trouble and eliminates it. At worst, these panaceas do definite harm; at best they are only a temporary alleviation.

In the last decade an immense amount has been done in the form of various types of publicity to inform the general public about proper nutrition and healthy diet, and it has borne amazing results in a drastically decreasing number of complaints of indigestion and constipation. But there is still too much trouble.

Indigestion and constipation may arise from countless causes, from organic stomach trouble, liver trouble, wrong diet—but it is being more and more realised that tension too plays a part. Whether the tension is mental, emotional or muscular, the effect is the same.

Constipation and Hæmorrhoids

We have discussed improved breathing habits as one effective means of getting rid of tension. We have learned that proper muscular function of the lower back, abdomen and buttocks helps. Now I want to give you another hint that has proved effective in constipation as well as in relieving hæmorrhoids.

Where constipation is caused by tension around the rectum, a good way to relieve it is to stand with your feet six inches apart and shake your knees, as you have learned to shake your wrists and your ankles. Within a few minutes this will relieve the spasms in your rectum.

Another position that brings relief in constipation and is helpful in reducing hæmorrhoids is the following:

Stand with your toes turned in so that you are pigeon-toed and the toes touch. If you remain in this position for a few seconds, breathing deeply, it will relieve the tension in your rectum. In case of hæmorrhoids, this simple remedy should be tried several times a day. Be sure that while your toes touch your knees remain straight, without bending.

Hæmorrhoids are small blood tumours around the anal orifice. They are exceedingly painful and often burst, causing bleeding. They develop ordinarily because of tension, improper sitting habits and constipation, or weak blood-vessels. Sitting on flabby buttocks puts too much unnecessary weight on the end of your spine and your rectum.

Pull the buttocks together and sit on your thighs. In this position the rectum does not touch the chair, the lower back straightens out, and your thighs carry the weight of your body.

According to Dr. E. G. Wakefield of the Mayo Clinic, fatigue, failure to relax, and anxiety are present in all cases of functional disorders of the colon and these may be the sole factors responsible in the production of symptoms.

The Liver and Kidneys

Tension affects the liver because it interferes with the rhythmic flow of bile and causes congestion. In severe cases, tension may even be responsible for stones in the gall bladder. The same applies to the kidneys, particularly when tension settles in the back, preventing proper circulation around the kidney region.

Your Teeth and Your Emotions

"Oh, come," you say, "I'm willing to accept a lot, but I don't see how tension can affect my teeth."

And yet not long ago the New York *Herald Tribune* reported a dental meeting under the caption: "GUM DISEASES LAID TO EMOTION OF FRUSTRATION."

"Dentists' session," a sub-heading read, "is told trench mouth is among ills caused by tensions." Dr. Sol J. Ewen, a research assistant at the Presbyterian Medical Centre, pointed out at this meeting that the mind and the body cannot be taken as separate problems and that the teeth cannot be treated without regard to the patient as a whole—his emotions, his fears, his frustrations—as well as his cavities. He pointed out that gum diseases tend to follow the emotional make-up of the patient, that mild tension resulted in mild inflammation of the gums while acute tensions brought about acute attacks of Vincent's infection.

Allergies and Anxiety

Dr. William Grant Lewi has declared that asthma, hay fever, and other allergies are caused primarily by improper functioning of the nervous system. The same applies to many diseases of the skin, ranging from the "nervous rash" with which we are all familiar to more serious ailments.

132

Dr. W. Horsley Gantt, carrying on Pavlov's experiments, discovered that even dogs can develop anxiety neuroses and asthmatic breathing.

Headaches

There are many medical authorities who believe that migraine is a result of unreleased emotional tensions. A Headache Clinic established at Montefiore Hospital in New York City claimed that by helping headache sufferers with their emotional problems, they were able to cure over eighty per cent. The headache, Dr. Arnold P. Friedman reported, "is often a symptom, a signal of emotional tension. . . . In all [chronic headache] emotional factors play an important part in the frequency, duration and severity of the headaches."

The Eyes

There is one school of thought, sponsored by Dr. Bates, which believes that eye troubles are all a result of strain growing out of tensions. Certainly, there are on record innumerable cases of people who have become blind because of shock, worry, or fear, although the eyes themselves have remained perfectly normal.

Much publicity was given, not long ago, to the case of a forty-year-old landscape gardener who became totally blind. During the last war he was emotionally upset because of the enormous destruction of trees, flowers, and growing things, which as a naturalist he greatly loved. His sight faded until he became blind. After a period of readjustment during which he learned to be self-supporting, his emotional tensions began to relax and with them the muscular tensions. His sight returned and there is no reason, according to his doctors, to believe that he need lose it again.

The Prevention of Disease

All of the foregoing sums up to the conclusion that tension

133

can affect every part of the body and play a part in almost every malady. You begin to see, therefore, a situation which should have immensely cheering factors for you. Because you realise that, if you master the art of relaxation, if you re-train your body in its habits, you can prevent a great many of the ills to which the flesh is heir. That you can, in effect, stay well and live longer. You are not a helpless victim. Far from it. Tension is preventable and tension is curable.

And speaking of prevention, the best way of all is to budget your energy as you budget your income. Learn to know how much you can do, how long it should take you, how fast you can do it. Then live within your income. An uncle may die and leave you a fortune, but no one can add an extra day to your life.

Learn how to stop *before* you are fatigued, to release your tensions, to rest not because you are prostrated but as a precaution. You can add years to your life this way and carry on under the most strenuous conditions without fatigue.

You will learn, too, if you arrange an intelligent energy budget for living (see chapter on "How to Live on Twenty-four Hours a Day") that you will acquire that fountain of youth for which the world is seeking. Fatigue, nervousness, tension and irritability all leave their marks upon you in lines and pouches in the face, in the tense expression that ages you.

The well person, the happy person, looks as though his face had been "ironed out". His friends look at him and say, 'You look years younger! What has happened to you?'

And the wise person replies, "Something important has happened. I have learned how to live."

CHAPTER ELEVEN

How to Prevent Tension in Children

ONE question that comes up again and again is, "When do the bad habits start that lead to tension?"

Unhappily, tension frequently has its root in earliest childhood. We are learning now that much of delinquency, stuttering, inferiority, and embedded fears arise when children are surprisingly young; that tension often develops too early, not only causing a disruption of personal rhythm and a loss of a sense of security, but frequently retarding mental development. It is astonishing at any age, as a matter of fact, to see the increased mental alertness and concentration that come as a result of relaxation.

Look at the baby crowing in his crib, waving his arms and legs. This is the supreme example of complete breathing and relaxation. His body is in perfect alignment; all of the muscle groups are functioning fully and flexibly; he is breathing according to his own personal rhythm. His changes from unhappiness to happiness, from smiling to tears, occur in a few seconds, revealing nature's wonderful harmony in balancing moods.

What are the disturbances that alter his personal rhythm, restrict his breathing, and create muscular tensions?

Sitting Up Too Soon

Often enough, the disturbance starts when the baby is only a few months old and his proud parents are eager to have him sit up as soon as possible. When a child is allowed to follow his own instinct, he will sit up as soon as he feels that his muscles are strong enough to support him. The impatient parents hurry this development, with the result that the spine is often weakened and impaired, while the child not only loses his own instinct for balance and alignment, but also the sense of security that comes with doing what he is equipped to do. Anxiety complexes in grown-ups are frequently a result of muscular weaknesses which cause a feeling of insecurity.

The same happens in regard to walking. Many children like to crawl for a long time. When they are ready to stand on their own feet they will do so, but they should be allowed to crawl as long as they enjoy it, as crawling develops muscle groups that they will need for walking.

Sometimes children are rushed into walking too early with the result that they have weak foot muscles from the first step.

The trainers of racehorses are wise enough not to hurry their training. The colts are allowed to run free until they have had a chance to develop, and their bones and muscles are strong enough for training. We should apply this method with our children, letting nature do its own work—which it does superbly when it has no interference—and starting the training when the child is ready for it.

The Right Shoes

Now comes the important question of the first walking shoes. They should have soft soles but give some support around the ankles. Why soft soles? Does not the child need the support of a hard surface? No, and again no! If we all grew up wearing soft soles for the first years of our lives, not only would we have stronger feet but we might even escape many of our mental difficulties.

The importance of strength and right function in feet and legs cannot be stressed enough for both physical and mental health. By giving an infant a shoe with a hard leather sole, we prevent the muscles in the bottom of his feet from developing and moving as they should, and check the development of nerve sensations. The stiff leather holds the foot in place without flexibility, prevents him from grasping things with his toes—all the movements that are essential if the small foot is to develop strong and healthy.

I have observed the contrast between children who grew up wearing leather soles and those who had worn soft soles for the first few years, and the difference was remarkable. The children who had worn the soft soles climbed and jumped, they were fearless and full of self-confidence. When they climbed over rocks, their feet instinctively curved and caught hold. When they jumped, their ankles were so flexible that they bent, protecting them from muscle strain and offering pleasant insurance against future headaches.

Sandals Versus Soft Shoes

But sandals, many mothers insist, are just as good as soft shoes. Well, sandals are an improvement on the average shoe because they allow the foot to be aired and keep it from perspiring. But because sandals have hard soles they are still not the perfect footwear for small children. Adults, as well as children, are aware of the immense comfort that comes from soft bedroom slippers that permit free movement of toes, soles of the feet, ankles. In time, women may be wise enough to realise that the comfort and sense of well-being that come from soft shoes with cushioned inner soles are more important than the so-called fashion of the spike heels.

Preventing Flat Feet

The time to prevent flat feet is from the very beginning. Watch your child as he moves and crawls and breathes and takes his first steps. If he is not functioning properly, find out what is wrong. A good many parents say, "Oh, well, my father has a tendency to flat feet. It runs in the family. I suppose my child inherited it." Such parents are amazed to discover that at least eighty per cent of such cases can be corrected of the proper sense of body alignment and balance is established so that the child learns how to work correctly.

Developing Strong Legs

A boy of five was brought to my office because he walked clumsily and, when out of doors, playing and running around with other children, he had a tendency to fall more often than was normal.

I discovered that his feet were weak and that his sense of insecurity came from under-developed thigh muscles. Because he lived in a block of flats where there were lifts, he had never used his legs for climbing stairs. This situation is so common in cities that some kindergartens now teach children how to climb stairs.

Before putting the little boy to work, I massaged the nerve points of the thigh muscles and around his knees and joints to awaken the nerve sensation, and then I worked out a game that was more strenuous for me than for him but which had fine results. This was a hunting game and ended by my chasing him up and down several flights of stairs. He loved it.

Gradually I increased the pace to give him confidence and help him forget the many falls that had left him with a feeling of insecurity. To strengthen his ankles, I taught him to jump, first from a footstool, then a chair, then the steps of a ladder, and finally from my grand piano, which, for his size, was quite a jump.

All the small children on whom I tried these graduated jumping exercises got great benefit out of them, not only physically but psychologically as well. Parents are sometimes hard to convince that the jumping is not dangerous for their children but that it provides a wonderful means of developing self-confidence.

Later on, the mother of my little pupil reported that he had spent an active summer, had gained full balance, and that he joined the other boys in sports and held his own.

The way to guard against tension and habits that cause an improper muscle function is to watch your child closely, not only to see how he moves, but to understand what his own rhythm is. Mothers are great sinners in regard to disturbing the child's own rhythm. They drag him along at their own adult pace, not his. *Never rush a child.*

One of the most instructive ways of studying your child is to watch him while he is asleep. You will be amazed how much you will discover in this way. Restlessness and impaired breathing, mouth breathing instead of nose breathing, talking in his sleep, are a few of the things that will show up. Just sit quietly in the room without a light and get to understand your child.

Palate Correction

You may observe that your child has difficulty in concentrating, or gets dizzy on a merry-go-round, or develops hearing difficulties. In many of these cases, the trouble may be due to a palate that is formed too high and therefore causes pressure on arteries and veins, affecting the circulation in certain lobes of the brain and setting up tension.

Modern orthodontia can correct this malformation and bring about complete cures. Children who have had this palate malformation corrected lose their dizziness while swinging, concentrate without difficulty—the trouble is always more noticeable in arithmetic—and regain perfect hearing. *It is important, however, that the work should be done before the child is fifteen.*

Eye and Ear Defects

In many cases where children are considered slow in their work, unable to keep their minds on their studies, and too nervous for their age the trouble lies in ear or eye defects that have gone unnoticed. The earlier such conditions are remedied, the better for the child's well-being and his adjustment.

Bad Children Are Sick Children

Not long ago, a teacher who had devoted over fifty years to working with problem and delinquent children pointed out that in the overwhelming majority of cases the root of the delinquency was tension brought about by physical handicaps which the parents had been too indifferent, too ignorant, or too impoverished to correct.

Obvious physical handicaps, such as deafness, a disfiguring scar, a speech defect, arouse ridicule in other children and a feeling of frustration in the handicapped child, who either develops a sense of inferiority and defeat or, in his attempt to compensate for his handicap, "to show them", tries to express himself in anti-social ways because he cannot do so according to the social pattern.

In many cases, the physical handicap may have a much less obvious cause. It may lie in tensions created by a spinal defect which is not noticeable to the eye and hence is unsuspected by parents and teachers. In a single classroom in New York City, over sixty per cent of the children were found to have some spinal defect, only an infinitesimal percentage of these disorders being previously known to exist. Tensions of this kind are dangerous because they can throw the physical, mental, and emotional nature into disequilibrium with a resulting personality distortion and delinquency. *These are not bad children; they are sick children.*

Night Terrors

Another thing that appears, even at an early age, is symptoms of night terrors. Dr. Joseph Collins pointed out that:

"Night terrors are encountered at every age of childhood; they may be visited upon few-months'-old babies or upon children fifteen and sixteen years of age. Most generally they attack children of six to seven. . . . The commonest cause of night terrors is improper feeding. They may herald disequilibrium of the nervous system.

"The diagnosis is more difficult when night terrors happen in children apparently in good health who suffer from no fever, no digestive disorder, no apparent organic lesion of the nervous system. Parents who attempt to combat night terrors without consulting a physician do their child a profound disservice."*

Night terrors frequently appear in adolescents as well as young children, and too often pass unnoticed. The bewildered adolescent is apt to have learned that his parents adopt an attitude either of amusement or impatience in regard to his emotional turmoil and he learns to say little about it, in self-protection.

A wise mother will make a point of watching her adolescent child sleep from time to time—*without letting the child know that she has done so*—to see whether the sleep is undisturbed or whether the child is restless and nervous.

Another point that should concern the mother is the young child's habit of enuresis (bed-wetting). According to Alfred Adler, this habit, if it persists beyond infancy, is a result of some tension from which the child is suffering. Frequently, the child may feel that he has lost his mother's interest. It is, in however unpleasant a form, a means of calling the mother's attention to him.

The Child's Own Rhythm

Once you have learned by your observations what your child's rhythm is, try to keep it undisturbed. The mother who drags her child along, its short legs running to keep up with her, is doing the child a great disservice. She is creating tensions. At times she unwittingly causes a stubborn streak

*Insomnia, How to Combat It, Joseph Collins, M.D. Appleton-Century-Crofts, 1930.

to develop in the child; for stubbornness is often a child's reaction to a feeling of hopelessness in the face of grown-ups' lack of comprehension or their exorbitant demands.

The youngster who has been dragged along will come home tired and cross. The child who is taken out in a stroller and then allowed to play freely when he reaches a park, develops a sense for unhurried movement that later will show its results in his natural rhythm in sports.

Walking in a crowd is apt to cause fatigue and bring little refreshment. You can see this in most small children who love activity but are tired and plaintive after an extended walk on city streets. The noise, the jostling, the rush, all tend to make them nervous and fretful although they themselves are unaware of what is wrong.

You can observe the difference for yourself. Watch a child playing in a park where he can move at ease, unrestricted and in his own rhythm. His movements are purposeful; he has the freedom that comes with following his own rhythm; he is refreshed and stimulated. Now watch him hustle along the street at his mother's rhythm. There is no freedom of movement, only strain and anxiety. He is quickly tired.

Do Not Frighten Children

Now that we know how early in life fear complexes can have their root, when every adult knows of the torture that he has suffered at some time in his life from fear of one kind or another, it hardly seems necessary to warn parents not to create fear. And yet there are still too many parents who use fear as an unscrupulous weapon against their child—fear of black men, fear of the policeman or the doctor, fear of the dark, fear of excessive punishment—whether or not they intend really to inflict it. Stammering, as I point out later on, frequently is a result of sudden shock and fear.

The greatest help that any child can have to enable him to grow up balanced and healthy is *a strong sense of security.*

This is his bulwark against the world. Take that away from him and you leave him half-defeated at the outset.

During the last war, when millions of children were subjected to the hideous mental, emotional and physical strain of bombing, it was discovered that the children who were strongly conscious of their mothers' support and protection were able to endure an incredible amount of strain without material damage, while children who lacked this security suffered in countless ways.

Breathing and Emotional Control

In Italy I watched the effective way in which many mothers handled their children. They would tell the screaming or fractious or stubborn child to kneel beside them and say the Lord's Prayer. The child would start to say the familiar words, and little by little his crying or panting breath would quiet down because the prayer forced the child to control his breathing. When the prayer was finished, the child was calm enough so that he could listen quietly to what was said to him.

What applies to the single child applies equally well to children in groups. If teachers and parents were aware of the tremendous gain of knowing about breathing control and the effect of sudden breath changes in keeping discipline, this knowledge would be taught in all colleges.

The Surprise Principle

One of the most effective means of controlling children is by use of the surprise principle. How does it work? Well, a teacher enters her classroom to give an examination. She is aware, the moment she closes the door, that something is in the air. A certain restlessness and lack of discipline can be sensed. She realises that with the children so keyed up, it will be hard to get them to write a good test.

Suppose that she tries the unexpected. Instead of starting

the test, she talks about the match that is ahead, or a film she has seen, anything that will catch the attention of the group. What happens? Instead of shifting around restlessly, the class listens. Why? Because her words are unexpected and force them to listen. That means that they inhale and unconsciously hold their breath, are calmed down and concentration is restored. After five minutes of this, the test can be given to a quiet, attentive class.

In various forms, the surprise principle can be used again and again. It will always work. It saves punishment; it saves wear and tear on your nervous system and the child's; the child is grateful because you make him feel less ill at ease. The same idea works in reverse when children are tired and listless, rousing them to fresh energy.

Improving Your Child's Posture

Posture difficulties develop at an appallingly early age. One main reason for this is that children, particularly in cities, are shut in crowded quarters where they are not allowed the full exercise and development of their bodies. This causes more far-reaching harm than just under-developed muscles. The body, the mind, and the emotions should develop as one harmonious whole if we are to have a truly balanced personality. It is normal, healthy, and right that a child should have complete freedom and space for play.

One Sunday afternoon in winter I walked along West End Avenue in New York City. That is a residential avenue lined with high apartment buildings. Suddenly I stopped to watch two charming little girls, about eight years of age, beautifully dressed, rolling happily along the pavement in the snow. The passers-by watched in amazement. The sight of well-dressed children rolling down the pavement was a rare sight in the city.

I could imagine their small, crowded apartment far up in one of those buildings, and I understood why those strong, healthy youngsters were rolling so joyously in the snow. They

144

simply had to discharge energy and it was impossible to do so indoors. As I walked away, I began to calculate the amount of repressed energy in our city children, and it occurred to me that millions spent now on provision for adequate outdoor play for city children might save future millions in the building and maintenance of mental hospitals.

Instead of running, playing, developing their muscle groups, children, even before kindergarten, when they are in nurseries, start bad muscle habits by too much sitting. There should be more time spent in playing on the floor, where the back and legs can get a good work-out.

At the age of five, the law requires compulsory school attendance of children. This, in most cases, means many hours a day of sitting. Strong children are unlikely to be affected but the more delicate ones, whose dorsal muscles are weaker, soon tire of sitting upright. They are apt to assume an habitually bent posture, causing pressure in the internal organs and, in time, damaging respiration.

Country children, left to their own devices, stretch out full length in a meadow, doing nothing, watching the clouds drift by, or a bird, or a flower, or the swaying branches of a tree.

A child's instinct to play, sitting on the floor, or to read, lying full length on the rug, is natural and wholesome. But he learns to curb it when he hears his mother say in exasperation, "How many times have I told you to get off the floor. Sit in a chair. Straighten up! You're all bent over."

What's Wrong with Physical Education

Physical education, as it is often taught to-day, is based on the ancient ideas of building physical strength. Greek physical education was of this type. The mediæval tournaments had this purpose. The old system of gymnastics was planned with this reason in mind. The goal was precision and toughness, not relaxation and harmony of movement, and individual body development. The only alternative is organised games and sports, in which the theory seems to be that an entire school

145

will derive some physical benefit from seeing a dozen or so of their fellows in action. Even the participants are less likely to achieve a well-developed body than they are to acquire tense muscles, partial development with attendant imbalance, and a weakening of the heart (athlete's heart), instead of a preparation for endurance through life. *To educate a nation to any form of tension is dangerous.* We know the influence of tension on the mind. Tension is always looking for an outlet and this outlet may well be brutal and aggressive. Most children at the end of their gym periods feel exhausted instead of being relaxed and exhilarated.

None of this has any real relation to physical education, to teaching boys and girls what their bodies are, how they function, how to make them function rightly so that they can last a lifetime without breaking down. You have to take driving lessons and get a licence to drive a car. You start to drive your body in a state of appalling ignorance.

It is preposterous that we spend twelve to sixteen years educating the mind of a young person and send him out in the world with a body of whose workings he knows almost nothing. He is barely aware of the interrelation of his organs; he is not as clearly or as thoroughly informed as he should be in regard to sex—and the amount of anxiety and hidden fears caused by this ignorance is heartbreaking. He does not live so as to get the most out of his body and mind and emotions. He does not know how to avoid exhaustion and fatigue, those great modern enemies, which are due to his own improper functioning. He does not know the possibilities or guess at the resources of his own personality or his creative urges. Through popular books he acquires a superficial idea of this personality of his—superficial, because it deals only with outward manifestations. This view of personality as being represented by social mannerisms is as unreal as it would be to regard beauty from the standpoint of cosmetics alone. The personality is the sum total of your attributes, balanced and fully developed and completely expressed. *Your* attributes, remember.

The child is taught facts and skills, but he does not learn

how to use them to his best ability because he is not taught how best to use his energy, how to keep his mind fresh and keen and his spirits high and his confidence strong. He is not taught that his own security, like his strength, must come from within himself or how to draw on it. He is not taught that he can be a fully rounded personality only if body and mind and emotions are in balance. He is not taught, finally, how to take it when the blows begin to fall.

"And yet," his disappointed parents say "he did so well at school. I don't see what went wrong."

A New Approach

I believe that we under-estimate one factor—namely, the effect of purely physical well-being and a sensation of vitality in giving people the courage to take risks and to stand up under disappointment or difficulties. Too many young people to-day are dragging along, feeling tired out, without the surplus energy they need to tackle new things, to face challenges, to meet the future with hope. Fatigued people will look for security, they will look for easy jobs that will bring them protection in case of sickness and provision for old age, because they do not have enough faith in their own energy to rely on it to carry them through.

Fatigue is the greatest enemy of self-confidence. That explains the astonishing and comparatively quick results in changing and liberating the personality that come from proper training in breathing and relaxation as daily living habits.

"Happiness," said Holbrook Jackson, "is a form of courage." But happiness can come only to the relaxed, the rested, the balanced person. It is not an unattainable dream; it is not the pot of gold at the end of the rainbow. It is the magnificent gift we can help our own children to attain by teaching them the infinite potentialities of their own bodies, of their muscles and their nerves, which, in the long run, are their chief armour against the slings and arrows of outrageous fortune.

CHAPTER TWELVE

What Are You Afraid Of?

ACCORDING to Webster, the definition of "frustrate" is "to prevent from attaining a purpose, to balk, to bring to nothing, defeat, baffle".

For our purposes, we are going to consider frustrations as emotional results of an inferiority complex because, as we pointed out in the beginning of this book, we create our own frustrations. We do so because of the attitude of mind we adopt toward life and, as we have already learned, our mental, emotional, and physical conditions react constantly upon one another. It appears, therefore, that the key to the elimination of our frustrations lies in acquiring the techniques of relaxation that help us to overcome our sense of inferiority, which is at the core of our frustrations.

A sense of inferiority is almost universal, whether people wear it like a placard or whether they conceal it. It is not necessarily an evil. Like tension itself, it can make or mar. And back of most inferiority, with its crippling sense of inadequacy, lurks man's worst enemy—fear.

Fear

Fear lies at the root of nearly all the emotional difficulties that trouble mankind. An enormous literature has appeared in which attempts are made to teach people how to eliminate fear, shyness, anxiety, frustrations, and all those related emotions. But if we are courageous enough to face the truth, we must admit that we can never entirely eliminate fear. We must expect it as a part of our emotional existence. What we can do is to learn how to cope with it from early childhood so that it will not overwhelm us and make us so tense that we have no escape from it.

What we must learn at the outset is to analyse our fears, to find out whether they have a real or an unsound basis. As the effect on us is the same, it is frequently difficult for us to discover whether the fear is merely a mental, emotional, or physical habit we have acquired, or whether it is founded on a real condition.

Let us examine some of the common fears that trouble mankind. It is important to learn at the outset that you are not the only victim of your hidden fears. *You are never alone with them.* There are millions suffering from the same fear, the same worry, the same shame or guilt. Knowing that your experience is shared by countless others may help you to cope with your particular problem.

Fears in Childhood

Fears too often raise their ugly head while the baby is still in his cradle. Some authorities claim that the only fears with which a child is born are those of falling and of a loud noise; others appear within a short time unless the parents are alert to check the first symptoms. Unhappily, the parents are often to blame, sometimes from carelessness, sometimes from indifference or harshness, which breed a sense of emotional insecurity, sometimes because of their sheer stupidity in deliberately engendering fear in the child as a means of enforcing obedience.

A fear that looms large in childhood is a fear of parents. Many well-meaning parents would be shocked to know that they have set up real fears in their children, not through such overt means as harsh punishments, but through a form of strictness that was designed solely for the child's good, or by a lack of understanding of the child's point of view which created an impassable barrier between parents and child.

Many children of school age have told me that they were happy only at school, that they dreaded having to go home. In some cases they were afraid that their mother's unpredictable temper would lead to an outburst of scolding, although they would not know for what they were being punished. In other cases, they were unhappy because a brother or sister received all the affection and they felt unloved and completely left out.

In such cases, the lack of emotional security at home left physical marks in the form of tension. The children either became overbearing in an attempt to compensate for home neglect by establishing their importance at school, or they developed inferiority complexes. Frequently, they themselves were astonished when their physical troubles were traced back to these childhood experiences.

A young woman was constantly in financial difficulties because she could not keep her clothes budget straight. She always bought more clothes than she could afford. We found out that, being the sixth child in a large family, she had resented wearing her older sisters' old clothes all the years while she was growing up. She had always been conscious that her schoolmates observed her shabbiness. Because she felt at a disadvantage she subconsciously attempted in later years to make up for it by the number and variety of her clothes. When she realised why she was so extravagant, she was able to remedy the situation and cut down her reckless buying.

In another case, a girl came to me in great tension. We traced the trouble to an overwhelming fear of the dark that had started in her childhood. This was an emotional fear and there was no point in saying firmly, "There's nothing to be afraid of. Just relax." Instead, I advised her to make a habit of carrying a small flashlight around with her. As long as she knew that she could dispel the darkness whenever she wished, there was no occasion for the fear, and she began to get relief from tension.

Often these hidden fears, whose root lies back in childhood, grow out of some physical weakness that prevented the child from taking part in games and sports. Frequently, weak feet that prevented children from running and jumping normally, created tensions that inhibited movement and gave the child a feeling of distrust of himself. The change to self-confidence that follows the re-education of the feet is often unbelievable.

Fears in Adolescence

A common fear in the adolescent, which often settles physically in the form of muscular tension, is the fear of not making good, of not being as gifted as a brother or sister. This fear is rarely mentioned to anyone else. The child hides his doubts about himself, represses them, and they settle so deep that when the time comes to choose a profession, the young man or woman is secretly afraid to choose the one he really wants because of a sense of indaequacy, and therefore becomes one of the many, many thousands who simply "take a job".

We have all seen these people in their late thirties or middle forties when they discover that they are profoundly dissatisfied with their lives, that their occupation bores them, that they get no satisfaction out of it, that life is slipping by without their ever having done what they really wanted to do.

Of course you can't do it until you try. What are you afraid of ? That you don't know enough about it ? But every human being who succeeded in the field you want to enter had to start where you are now—knowing nothing about it, and hence having no real estimate of his capacity to do it.

The disappointment and frustration that come from turning away from the work you love without a trial create tensions, but here there is a fine chance for the person to help himself. If this happens to be your case, dig down to the root of your disappointment. Find out what hidden wish you have buried so deep. If you cannot now make it your occupation or profession, at least you can make it your hobby. The person who says that it is too late is creating an alibi for himself.

It is never too late. People have begun studying medicine in their forties and Greek in their seventies. If you approach your hobby with enthusiasm and joy, pouring into it all the creative quality that has been thwarted in the wrong channels, you will find your life enriched. How often people become experts in their hobbies and continue to reap a rich reward from them long after they have given up their bread-and-butter jobs.

Another common anxiety in teen-agers is the stirring of religious doubts. For the youngster who can talk out his problem, there is little difficulty. The one who hides it and worries about it begins to reproach himself with being bad and unworthy, and creates a state of mental and physical tension.

One young man told me about having struggled with religious doubts during his high school days. When he reached college, however, and heard other young men of his own age openly discussing their own doubts, the burden fell away. He realised that his was a common problem and that it was part of the process of growing up.

Superiority Through Smallness

At the root of an overbearing attitude, you will frequently find a deep-seated sense of inferiority with its embedded fears of inadequacy. The physically small person seems to be especially susceptible to this overbearing attitude in an attempt to compensate through power for lack of size. In these cases, the art of relaxation can change the whole attitude and therefore the whole life.

Such a case was that of a woman who was one of eight children. Prematurely born, she grew to only four feet eight inches. Though she was well proportioned, this tininess, among the group of brothers and sisters of average size, gave her a bad start from early childhood, especially as she had such weak feet that she was extremely timid of any form of physical exercise. At the age of eight, for instance, she was so terrified of jumping that it took her father hours to persuade her to jump down two steps.

The older she grew, the more she resented her smallness, particularly as the sister closest to her in age was both strong and good looking. In order to compensate for what she considered a misfortune, she became over-ambitious, domineering, and extremely tense.

Instead of trying to strengthen the weak feet which gave her a sense of physical insecurity, she wore high-laced shoes with arch supports. Instead of selecting clothes that would make her size attractive, she persisted in copying those of her sister, which were wrong for her. The relationship between the sisters inevitably became strained.

This bad start in early childhood later had its repercussions in the girl's professional life. Although intelligent and kind by nature, she developed such an overbearing, despotic attitude toward co-workers and later toward employees, that although she was respected she was always feared, a situation which eventually developed in her relationship with her own children also.

When she was about fifty, the effects of this long-accumulated tension became more than she could endure and she came to me for help. We started to release tension from her feet and legs and I explained that low-heeled shoes would give her far more rest than the high heels with which she tried to increase her height and only increased her tension. As she began to relax physically, she became a changed person emotionally, her relations with her family became warmer and the dominating quality dwindled away so that she was far easier to live with.

None of these difficulties need have arisen if she had learned as a child not to resent her size but to accept it and make the best of it, dressing in accordance with her own appearance and not with that of her sister.

Parents and teachers should be aware that the seemingly trivial tendency of a girl to copy the appearance of other girls or of film actresses, in a vain effort to make her personality like that of someone else, can do her infinite harm and that it is often the root of unreleased tension through life. Only the person who is completely himself can get real satisfaction out of life or make his personality attractive. Rubber-stamp personalities are uninteresting because they are unreal.

How Frustration Thwarts Talent

There was a young man of twenty-seven who wanted to be a commercial artist, but because of his muscular tensions he continually failed when he attempted to get a job in his own field.

I tried to find out what had caused these tensions in the first place and learned that as an adolescent he had worked in his father's store, although he did not like the job. His father was strict and did all he could to discourage the boy from taking up commercial art. Nothing that he did ever met with his father's approval and he was blamed for everything that went wrong.

At length, he realised that he had to get away from home and he came to New York, where he went to an art school. As long as he was at school, all was well with him, but when he started out to get a commercial art job the trouble started. All the frustration and discouragement to which he had been subjected began to take its toll. He had grown so tense that he could not stand up under any real physical effort, and, like most people who suffer from fears, he was particularly stiff in the intercostal muscles. No one looking for an employee would have considered him a good bet. He was neither physically fit nor did he give another person any feeling of confidence in his abilities.

I began to release the tension in the intercostal muscles and as soon as he could breathe deeply he began to feel more confident. We then took up the abused muscle groups one at a time until his body was erect and relaxed.

The next time he set out to look for a job, vigorous, alert, confident, he got the one he was after, and to-day he stands high in his profession with a national magazine.

Fear of Financial Insecurity

An unbalanced budget lies behind countless illnesses which

may appear on the hospital records as anything from heart disease and stomach ulcers to liver, gall-bladder and all the other diseases the flesh is heir to.

Constant worry and its accompanying fear about insufficient funds or old-age security or being able to meet the rent on the first of the month add up to overwhelming misery on the part of the people as a whole.

An immense percentage of all this worry stems from untidiness in money matters. Just as you avoid nervous strain by learning to be punctual in matters of time, so you can avoid much nervous strain, worry, and fear by finding out whether the root of your tension does not lie in a permanently upset budget.

Making ends meet is not a simple problem; it is difficult for most people. But, because it is difficult, they evade the issue and hope for the best and make no real effort to bring order to their financial affairs. And yet that initial effort is far simpler than the attendant strain that comes of knowing—with a knowledge that never really leaves you—that the problem is unsolved.

It is not the job of your physician to say, "Your trouble is a result of financial worry. Go home and sit down at your desk. Set down your basic expenses: rent, taxes, electricity, insurance, bus fare, laundry. Then see how much is left for food, clothing and entertainment. Get your budget in order. Once you have trained yourself to live within your budget, you will improve both in body and in mind."

Bed rest will not help if you have no mental rest. Pills will not cure financial worry. Exercises to relieve tension will not do the job of mental relaxation that comes with the meeting and solution of your problem. Perhaps this seems out of place in a book on the art of relaxation. But it is actually very much in place. Relaxing a muscle group is helpful, but we want to get at the core of your difficulties. If your basic problem is a fear of financial insecurity, that muscle group will not do enough for you. It will not release the nagging worry

155

in your mind, and worry accompanies an unsolved problem—not one you have solved.

How to Stop Worrying About Money

You may find out that, with your present expenses, you simply cannot balance your budget. In that case, it is unrealistic, to say the least, to wait like Mr. Micawber for something to turn up. Find out where you are spending too much money and do something about it. Perhaps you will have to cut down on your rent in order to have more money for food. Perhaps you will decide that for a while you will have to spend more on clothes in order to build up a wardrobe and therefore you must cut out all entertainment.

If you deal with the situation, instead of worrying about it, you will find that this tidying of your money affairs will have a beneficial influence on your mood, your mind, and your body. It will relax you more than any exercises you could take. Even if you must restrict yourself to a far simpler life than the one to which you are accustomed, the recompense of having no money worry will pay in better health and sleep and spirits.

I have never heard more incessant talk about money worry than among the very rich who do not keep within their income, but I know many who live in peace of mind on a small income because they plan to spend in accordance with what they have.

This problem of financial security is one which the free-lance worker must face at the outset. He must realise clearly, in deciding on his profession, that—unlike the salaried worker—he cannot tell in advance how much money he will make, that his income will be irregular and, for the first years at least, hazardous. He must decide for himself whether his independence is worth this uncertainty. Once he has made his decision, he must not keep casting longing glances at the other side; he must accept the results. That is, if he has decided he prefers the security of the regular job, he will only arouse tensions and frustrations by longing for independence; if he

156

has decided on free-lance work, he must accept the risks as a necessary part of his choice and not keep longing for the security of the regular income.

Fear for the Family

A common fear of middle-aged parents, particularly the father of the family who shoulders the financial responsibility, is that he cannot provide for the future security of his family; that if he were to be ill, there is not enough money in the bank to keep his family going, provide an education for his children, and, particularly, to look after them when he is gone.

And this brings us to a subject that causes almost universal tension to-day—the search for security and the fear of insecurity. And it brings us to a point which an overwhelming number of people find themselves unwilling to accept. For I am not trying, in this book, to make wild and bright promises or to tell you that all is for the best in the best of all possible worlds. Earlier, I pointed out that we can never entirely eliminate fear but that we can learn how to cope with it. Now I must point out that the thing people call security has become in the modern atomic world an escapist's dream.

The anxious father, wanting to extend his financial protection over his children after his death, is aiming at the unattainable. In a shifting world, it is almost an impossibility to ensure the continued security, in a financial sense, of one's children. Storm and flood and hurricane; war and devastation and the wiping away of properties; bank failures; all these can shake or wipe out the soundest "protection".

The experiences of the past thirty years when kingdoms tumbled, countries vanished, and people by the hundreds of millions became homeless, even separated from one another, have proved the truth of this statement.

But just as we can learn to cope with fear, so the harassed parent can learn to provide his children with a different means of facing the fear of insecurity. That is, by teaching them to acquire the only real security there is, the inner strength that

157

comes with learning self-confidence, self-reliance, the ability to stand on their own feet rather than depend on the father's savings in an uncertain future; and, of course, the practical and concrete assistance that comes with training them by education for a job or profession which can support them in time of need.

Fears of the Wrong Weight

It is always a shock to realise how many lives are warped because people have grown increasingly conscious of their appearance, and the fact that they are too fat or too thin causes widespread misery. Much tension has developed simply because men and women are overweight or underweight.

There was a girl who came to ask if anything could be done to help her put on weight. She was so thin that it made her miserably self-conscious and she refused to go swimming, or to parties where she was expected to wear evening dress. Her embarrassment and self-consciousness had developed into a sense of inferiority and a growing tension. She had lost her appetite.

As soon as she understood that her salvation was to learn how to let go and take it easy and forget about her looks, thinking instead of how she felt, she began to improve. She gained weight as soon as she began to relax, her appetite came back, and as the muscles around her chest relaxed and she began to breathe correctly, she enjoyed life and took up social activities again.

The psychological effect of overweight may be judged by the torture which stout people are willing to endure to rectify the situation—the sweating, the pummelling, the rigid diets, all of which have bad effects on the general health.

In the case of overweight people, there is more involved than an unattractive appearance. For some reason, the fact of putting on weight gives people a feeling of guilt. They regard their weight as a sign of self-indulgence. Before attempting to work with the overweight, I first send them to their doctors for a check-up. It is interesting to see what happens to them when they learn, as they sometimes do, that their trouble comes from a glandular condition and not from excessive appetite or indulgence. Their self-respect comes flooding back. It is then easy to teach them to correct their wrong habits.

How to Overcome Boredom

Not long ago, Dr. Robert McCracken of Riverside Church in New York City devoted an entire sermon to the problem of boredom. Problem, you ask? Yes, indeed. For boredom is an emotion which not only causes a feeling of frustration but has physical effects as well. When you are bored, you feel listless, irritable, fatigued, without energy.

Boredom is, after all, simply a state of mind. It is not induced by outside circumstances. It is a result of your own attitude toward those circumstances. Life is interesting only if you take an interest in it. You can conquer boredom by the way in which you meet the challenge of every day, the way you regard the small events that can either pass unnoticed or end in interest, joy, and the building of new relationships.

Some years ago, at the time when zippers were just coming into use and frequently got stuck, a woman was on a train. Across the aisle there was an old lady who was trying in vain to open her zippered handbag. The woman, who was always interested in people around her, offered to help, a conversation began, and when they reached their destination the old lady extended a cordial invitation to the younger woman to visit her. Out of this conversation grew a real friendship and through the old lady the younger woman met people who, in times of adversity, enabled her to build a new existence. That was a lot to grow out of an active interest in a zipper that would not work.

You should teach yourself never to be bored. If you find yourself in a gathering where the activities and the conversation hold no possible interest for you, detach yourself and get your interest from watching the way people move, or the expressions on their faces, or the tones of their voices. Try to picture them as children or under other circumstances, and you will forget all about your boredom.

Fears in Middle-aged Women

The fears of women are twofold. The first is the hidden fear of nearly all women. It starts in the forties. That is the woman's fear of losing her looks because of age. Whatever her personal reason may be—whether she fears losing the love of her husband to a younger and more attractive woman, or fears losing her job because of age—this fear will grip her some day and hold her in its claws.

Beauty treatments, exercises, falsifying of age records are all well-known remedies. But no method will really be effective to the victim of age-fear itself, even though she may succeed in deceiving others.

A part of this fear is no longer necessary—and that is the fear of menopause suffering. Medicine has made giant strides in this direction, our knowledge of glands has increased almost overnight, and it is now possible for a woman to go through her menopause with far less physical or mental disequilibrium.

The fear of age itself is a different thing. Here your only remedy is to acknowledge to yourself that nothing can be done to prevent you from growing one day older every day. That is an inescapable fact. It is not a fact that touches you alone. It is the common fate of mankind. But once you have the courage to accept the fact that the sun goes down every night, even though you would sometimes like to prolong a good day, you can change your hidden fear into fun.

It all depends really on the point of view you adopt. Try to stay young, by all means, to look young and to feel young and to *be* young. But don't go at it as though you were furtively and shamefacedly adopting a disguise, as though you were trying to deceive those around you.

Play the game of staying young consciously and frankly. Accept it as a challenge and enjoy it. Of course you want to be young. Who doesn't? Make yourself look young. But you can't do that simply by taking beauty treatments. The signs of age are from within and they have to be attacked there. *Tension ages!* Learn to keep yourself flexible in body and mind and it will astonish you to discover how much younger you feel. It will surprise you, too, to learn how little age or looks matter in the woman who has a talent for being relaxed and flexible.

Looks, as a matter of fact, have always been less essential than women believe them to be. The great charmers have almost never been beautiful women; some of them have been downright ugly. Study the faces of the great actresses, of the women who are the most popular in any gathering, and you will realise that they are rarely beauties. Their attractions rest on vibrant personalities.

If you try to hide your age fear, it will do its destructive work secretly, making you tense and unpleasant. Look it in the face and accept it and you will begin to get more enjoyment out of every day. In time you will agree that it is not your age that counts but the pulsing content of everyday experience that makes up your life.

Any woman who can grow old with this courage will discover that what she loses in looks she gains in human relations. Young people instinctively make friends with older women who have the courage to act according to their age. Your own generation of friends will be kinder, because they often resent one of their own age group who tries to escape. Older people will gladly seek your company because to them you are still welcome youth.

A second fear that grips many women at about the age of forty is that of losing their jobs. Since the time of our grandfathers, life expectancy has increased by almost eighteen years, which means that this brand of fear has taken on new proportions and society has not yet learned to cope with it. There are two reasons for this: one is that there are more older people to-day than ever before in history; the second is that no adequate provision for those later years has been made.

These two fears that attack women in their middle years have a foundation in solid, inescapable fact. They are at the root of innumerable mental illnesses, and rob millions of women of peace of mind. The second fear is a problem for society to solve, because it concerns what, in increasing proportions, has become a form of mass anxiety. On the other hand, the first fear is a problem for the individual to tackle and solve for herself. It will always be the problem of the individual.

What a woman gets out of her later years will depend one hundred per cent on her own intelligent grasp of her problem and on her willingness to accept reality and to meet it gallantly.

Fears in Older Men

There are other fears that we all share, more or less, but that each one believes to be his or her own personal trouble. In men, it is largely the fear of having to retire at sixty-five, or of being unable to find a job when over fifty and being useless. Even in circumstances where the financial situation does not justify fear, because a living is provided for by insurance or a pension, the fear complex persists.

To grow old without fear and bitterness is perhaps the hardest job we have to accomplish in life. This, as we have noted, is a comparatively new problem, at least in its present proportions, when: "The average life expectancy is now 65.1 years for white males and 70.3 years for white females. . . . In other words, children born to-day have a life expectancy of about eighteen years beyond the age that could be claimed for their grandparents."

But we have not yet done much to provide for these added years. Retirements are still enforced at an age when many men feel that they have their full capacities and resent being deprived of their work.

Neither fear nor resentment can solve the problem. If every man would realise that his is not an individual but a human problem, he would be able to accept it more easily and to prepare for the time when he will have to give up his accustomed earning job. What do I mean by preparation? First, learning to face the situation. Instead of shying away from it, resenting it, fighting against the inevitable, pretending that the condition does not exist, you must learn to talk about it calmly, to look around for activities to fill up time and use energies when the day of retirement comes. Perhaps you will find that your former hobby can become a full-time occupation; perhaps you will serve on the committee of your favourite welfare organisation; perhaps you can move to the country and begin to cultivate your garden—and nothing gives a man a stronger sense of continuity than that.

Whatever course you decide upon, you should not allow yourself to become tense at the prospect of change and, through tension, resentful. There is so strong and inevitable a connection between physical and mental tension that everyone who really tries can prevent himself from turning into an elderly misanthrope.

CHAPTER THIRTEEN

How to Overcome Frustrations

FEARS, as we pointed out earlier, are an inescapable part of man's lot, but while he cannot entirely avoid them he can at least learn to cope with them intelligently; so that he is their master instead of becoming—as he too often does—their victim.

We owe one kind of unreleased tension through fear to our increasing civilisation and the code of manners and behaviour that accompanies it. The person who has self-control feels that he must, under all circumstances, refrain from betraying his feelings publicly. When asked how he feels, he holds up his head, smiles, and answers cheerfully, "I feel fine". His code demands that he do this even when he feels rotten, is secretly convinced that he has all the symptoms in the *Materia Medica*, and believes that he will probably lie down and die before evening.

Up to a certain point, this kind of behaviour is not only proper, it is almost indispensable. Everyone has so many burdens of his own that life would become intolerable if he were expected to shoulder all the aches and pains of his friends and neighbours. For the sake of his fellows, therefore, his restraint is admirable. For his own sake, however, it is not so good. He stores up a lot of complaints that settle in the form of tensions unless he gets rid of them.

Releasing Fear Through Action

Let us suppose, for instance, that you receive notice, like a bolt from a clear sky, that you have lost your job. You need the money urgently, not only for yourself but for those who are dependent upon you. At the same time you have sustained a bad shock. What do you do? Well, if you are a normal, civilised person, you hold your head high and smile at your co-workers.

Inside, however, you are gripped by fear of what will become of you and your dependents. The more you attempt to conceal your fear the harder it will work inside. What, then, are you to do?

Smile, by all means, as long as you are at your place of work, but bear in mind that you must allow yourself an outlet later on, and the sooner the better.

It is always a tremendous help if you can release nervous tension through action. If it is possible to do so, take a long walk and work that bad news out of your system by exercise. Try to do it the same day, so that the fear will not have an opportunity to settle in your system.

If walking is not practicable, go to a film that night so that your thoughts and tensions will be released through new emotions. Or, if you have an understanding friend, talk it out. Get it out of your system.

This is the healthy way to do it. The unhealthy way is the kind of restraint that makes you decide, "I'll keep it to myself". But the fear is there and the fear refuses to be ignored. If you don't walk it out or talk it out, it reacts upon the body. How many skin ailments and upset stomachs, violent headaches and bad colds could have been avoided if people had been aware that the tension must be released before it took its toll on the body!

Talking It Out

Talking it out is a sound method of releasing fear and stored-up tension. The old expression "Getting it off your chest" has a literal meaning. So long as the tension is there, the chest is actually oppressed by shallow breathing, and until that tension is released, you cannot get back to normal.

Naturally, I don't mean that you must go to the extreme of making a nuisance of yourself by turning the shoulder of every friend and acquaintance into a Wailing Wall. Nor have I much patience with the person who always takes the expression, "How are you?" as an invitation to describe his symptoms. But there is a middle ground.

Pick out a person who knows you and who will listen with sympathy and understanding. Then *acknowledge your fear.* Talk about it. It is the unacknowledged fear that grows out of control. The normal fear, when it has been looked at and dissected and analysed and probed, will begin to dwindle until it ceases to be a menace; it is simply a fact to be reckoned with.

Nearly every human being carries around with him some unacknowledged fear that colours his viewpoint and his actions; hampers his courage and his self-confidence. Suppose you search your own heart for such a fear. Is it based on your ignorance of some essential facts—such as a proper and sound knowledge of sex; is it a fear of some lack in yourself or the feeling that you have some bad habit that others neither have nor suspect in you? Is it a fear of people or of situations or of your environment or of your own inadequacy?

Don't Bury Your Fears

Whatever your fear, one thing is sure. It is not yours alone. That same fear lurks in a million other hearts. As long as you keep it buried, you walk in shackles. Take a good look at it in the light of day and then, for heaven's sake, talk about it! Once it comes out in the open, it is no longer a danger to you.

Sometimes this buried fear is concealed because of a mistaken consideration for others. There are people who learn from their doctors that they suffer from an incurable condition and that they cannot live long. To spare their family and friends, they say nothing, and bear the burden alone. But the price which they pay in unreleased tension in the long run levies its toll upon them and, often enough, upon the very people whom they were trying to spare.

How widespread the need to talk things out becomes has

166

been made apparent by the rise of Worry Clinics, whose only function is to provide sympathetic listeners. It is not their function to advise or even to comment. Simply to listen.

Talking aloud, although not so good as the interchange of ideas that comes with a frank discussion and give-and-take of opinion, has at least the advantage of crystallising the problem simply through the necessity of putting it into words. Frequently, just talking the situation out helps to clarify it and, by relieving nervous tension, helps the victim of the fear not only to see his own problems more clearly, but to be relaxed enough to cope with them. For—make no mistake about it!—the tense person never has the same amount of courage as the relaxed one.

Keeping Up a Front

Some time ago, I encountered an extreme example of self-restraint carried so far that the woman not only refused to betray her emotions to others, she would not even permit herself to express them when she was alone.

She was an exceptionally intelligent person, a widow of fifty, the mother of two grown sons and two daughters. She came to me because, she said, "I feel as though I would crack with tension". She was plagued with insomnia and her muscles were as stiff as though she had been encased in an iron ring. Perhaps, she said, I would be able to teach her how to sleep again.

She was a woman of infinite reserve and had built a life on emotional restraint. As we worked to limber up her muscles we talked. I discovered that although she loved her children and they gave her their deepest respect, it never warmed into affection. Even after the death of a husband whom she had adored, she would not permit herself to weep for him. Even for herself she had to keep up a front. And her body, of course, had taken its revenge for all those stored-up emotional tensions that should have been released in human expression.

As the muscles of her chest and shoulders began to relax,

I could feel her let go for the first time in her life. She wept and wept, as a result of that sensation of physical relief which brought with it an emotional relief. That night she slept. Insomnia, she discovered, was something she had been doing to herself. The cure lay not in a disciplined body but in a relaxed body.

Gradually, she learned how to let go, and as the physical rigidity relaxed, there was an unexpected emotional flowering. She not only lost her fear of cracking up and her insomnia, but she began to live more richly and had the delight of creating a new relationship with her children that was founded on human warmth and deep affection.

Tension—and few people realise this—creates an emotional block. The person who is "all tied up" is unable to experience emotions as deeply, as fully as he should.

What Fear Does to the Body

Over and over again, I have encountered the physiological results of fear that has been unreleased. I have discovered, for instance, that great tension is to be found in the intercostals—the muscles between the ribs—and particularly between the sixth and seventh ribs. As soon as this tension can be released physically, through complete breathing which makes the muscles flexible, the grip of fear is released.

In Florence, Italy, the director of a dancing school sent me a twelve-year-old girl who turned pale and became so dizzy after a few steps that she was unable to dance. Her family doctor could find no physioloical reason for her condition.

I watched her when she came in and said unexpectedly, "Tell me what gave you such a bad shock."

In her surprise, she poured out the story. She had been riding a bicycle along a lonely street a year before when a man had attempted to attack her. It was difficult to determine from her excited account whether the man's intentions had really been bad or whether the girl had misunderstood him because

168

—according to the custom of her country—she had rarely been alone on the street.

Whether or not the fear was justified, the shock was real. The child had been too frightened to tell anyone about it and the shock had settled in her system, giving rise to a bad breathing habit. She pulled up her diaphragm while she inhaled and thus blocked circulation. This pull of the diaphragm also caused a pressure against the heart. About eighty-five per cent of nervous people acquire it. Naturally, this had a bad effect as soon as she began to dance.

When I knew the source of the trouble and discovered the bad habit she had acquired, I was able to correct it in eight or nine lessons so that the child learned to breathe with a flexible diaphragm. She took up her dancing lessons without further difficulty. When her parents came to see me, they reported that not only had her appetite greatly improved but that she had become a much happier person.

Stammering

Stammering based on psychological causes can easily be cured through restoration of the disturbed breathing rhythm.

I remember the case of a four-year-old boy in the country in Germany. In the course of a few days he developed a bad stammer and his mother traced the cause to shock. A chimney sweep had appeared suddenly before the child after he had finished his work. The sight of the black man had so frightened the boy that he began to scream. Within a few days the stammering started and rapidly grew worse.

Once I knew the cause, the cure was easy. When the chimney sweep came the next time, I met him and explained the situation. He was the father of several children, a kindly and understanding man, and he was willing to help. When his work was done, he came out of doors where the mother was waiting with her small boy at her side.

At the sight of the black man, and remembering his former shock, the child became frightened. But the chimney sweep, holding in his outstretched hand some candy with which I had provided him, walked toward the child and began to talk casually.

Slowly the small hand reached out and the child accepted the candy. As the chimney sweep continued to talk, the boy started to laugh, and eventually he dared to touch the man and lost his fear. We repeated the cure a second time and the stammering disappeared because the fear was released.

The same result can be obtained when the stammering has become a habit of years' standing. A twenty-year-old girl from Scotland stammered badly as a result of fright when she was seven years old. It had happened, she said, when her brothers were playing ghosts and suddenly invaded her nursery, wrapped in white clothes and emitting blood-curdling howls. The terrified child developed a bad stammer.

We discovered the consonant combinations that made her stammer. Instinctively she tightened up whenever she was about to pronounce them. I explained to her what she did to her diaphragm by this tightening habit, and after working hard at strenuous exhaling and whistling to relax the diaphragm, we began to tackle the frightening consonant combinations while she was relaxed. We kept at them until she enjoyed rather than feared saying them, and she freed herself of her thirteen-year-old habit of stammering.

How to Get Rid of Frustrations

One day the wife of a prominent executive came to see me. Was there, she asked pleadingly, anything that could be done to improve her appearance? With every movement, with the tone of her voice, with her walk and the carriage of her head, she betrayed an inferiority complex. Even her walk was insecure. She looked as though she was trying in vain to excuse herself for existing.

As I had met her overbearing husband, it was not difficult to discover the reason for the condition in which she found herself. A problem like this cannot be tackled without a strong awareness of the fact that the mind and the body are inter-related, that they influence one another. The attitude of the mind can, in the long run, influence the carriage of the body, while posture has a direct and an immediate effect on the state of mind. William James pointed out long ago that we do not run because we fear; we fear because we run. We begin to cringe because we are warped by a feeling of inferiority; then we feel more and more inferior because we cringe. It is, you see, a vicious circle.

Well, we had to start somewhere. There did not seem to be any practicable way of remaking her husband but at least we could counteract his effect on her. As she stood looking at me, it was apparent that she was in no condition to cope with arrogance. She could only succumb to it.

Muscular tensions vary with every individual, but after reading the earlier chapters, in which we have traced the various muscle groups, you are in a position now to know where your tensions lie. In this particular case, the lower back region was weak, and the bowed head was due to stiffness in the shoulders and neck.

We began with breathing, bringing all the muscles of the shoulders into play, retraining the neck to stand upright on flexible muscles, creating new posture habits as the back grew stronger. As the muscles gained in flexibility, her posture improved. The increased intake of oxygen through deeper breathing not only made her feel better but made her feel more self-reliant. As her posture improved, so did her per-spective.

A spring came back into her walk, she entered a room with poise and self-confidence; her voice, which had been muted, a mere apologetic whisper, was full and clear. She had become a personality.

Not long ago I saw her again, a changed woman. But the change had gone far beyond the surface improvement, al-though she laughed with pleasure as she repeated to me the compliments she was constantly receiving on her appearance.

The incredible thing, she said, was that she no longer trembled like Sweet Alice at her husband's frown. And her husband had come, imperceptibly but increasingly, to turn to her for her opinion and judgment, and to depend on her.

To see frustrations give way to a sense of fulfilment is the most rewarding thing I know. The heart-breaking factor is that it could happen in thousands and tens of thousands of cases, if people would only realise to what an extent they cause their own frustrations and foster their own sense of inferiority. The cure lies with them and with it the full flavour of life, instead of the flatness for which most of them settle because of sheer inertia.

Unsolved Emotional Problems

One day an elderly business woman came to me to learn how to relax. Tension was not only making her physically miserable but distorting her emotional attitudes so that her relationships not only with her business associates but also with her friends and her immediate family had become strained and difficult.

While she was lying down, I watched her tense face with lines etched by hidden fears, and asked abruptly, "What frightened you as a child?"

When she made no reply, I asked again, "Was it your father or your mother?" This was, frankly, a shock method, but it is useful because its surprise leads almost always to a truthful response, while more preparation simply builds resistance.

"How did you guess?" she asked.

"I didn't guess," I explained. "There is an expression of fear on your face, so deep-rooted that it must go far back in your life."

The tension, as she poured out the story, could be traced back to a tyrannical mother who had aroused bitter opposition in her daughter but at the same time had left her with such a sense of frustration that she did not know how to free herself of the despotism. The unreleased tension had played a

172

part in breaking up her marriage and later had led to unhappy relations with her children. Without realising it, she was subjecting them to much the same type of despotism that had victimised her as a girl.

Like many women with unsolved emotional problems at home, she threw herself into her business life with terrific energy. Women of this type appear to justify themselves by thinking, "I am working so hard that no one can expect anything more of me".

The net result of unreleased tension, emotional conflict, and overwork was that she was in extremely bad health and on the verge of a breakdown.

My first task was to get at the cause, of which she herself had been unaware—in this case, the frustrations and tensions growing out of an oppressed girlhood. When she herself understood what was wrong, she was willing to co-operate.

The next step was to show her that she had to keep her energy budget balanced. One day a week must be set aside for rest and recuperation. She was to consider that day non-existent. No appointments were to be made. No household chores were to be left for that free time. She was to stay in bed, reading if she liked, or simply resting. Her food was to be prepared the day before so that she would not spend time bustling around and getting it.

The first day of bed rest was a trial. She was not used to inactivity. She felt guilty about it. She wanted to get up and do the small things she had forgotten. But she stayed there. The next week it was easier. Within a month it was a habit she took for granted.

By the end of a few weeks she discovered that the tensions in her business life were beginning to disappear. When she relaxed, the people around her became less antagonistic. They relaxed, too. Much of the strain of her work fell away and she began to enjoy it instead of worrying about it.

Best of all, her relations with her children improved. Aware of her own tense manner, she began to change her habits, she no longer attempted to dominate her children, and they began to come to her spontaneously with the confidences she had formerly demanded of them.

Overcoming a Sense of Inferiority

The shoulders provide an excellent index to one's sense of inferiority. The deep sigh of relief that people heave as their shoulders become flexible not only has physical value but it causes a mental and emotional relief. Tense shoulders cause repressed energy that has a bad effect both on the organs and on the brain.

Observe any person with stiff shoulders. How repressed he looks! Try it yourself and see what it does to you; it takes away your feeling of vitality, your self-confidence, and restricts your whole outlook.

What causes this sense of inferiority? We have been hearing a great deal about it and people still regard it as some kind of personal attribute with which one is born, like red hair.

Nonsense. An inferiority complex seems to be a part of man's heritage. The man who blusters or the Caspar Milquetoast—at the heart of almost everyone there is a certain element of this sense of inferiority. The problem is how to deal with it. There are three ways of tackling the problem. One is to give up the battle because you are inferior to it; one is to escape from reality by any one of a number of methods—daydreaming, liquor, and other devices—and pretend that the problem does not exist. The third is to study the situation, estimate why you feel inferior and to what you feel inferior, and then try to rectify the situation.

If you belonged to the first category—the one that is willing to submit without a struggle—you would not be reading this book. If you belong to the second category, you probably hope that in these pages you will find a magic formula that will change the situation for you without effort. But let's go on the theory that you belong to the third category. You are shackled by a sense of inferiority and you are determined to get the better of it.

174

A sense of inferiority, like tension, is not an evil in itself. Just as tension can prove to be an agreeable sensation and accompany the great moments of our lives, so a sense of inferiority can become, and indeed has been, the impetus behind our advance in civilisation, in humanity, in the codes that have raised us in moral stature and created beauty around us.

But the sense of inferiority is useful only when it leads us to overcome it.

As we have pointed out before, the task that you fail to perform or leave half finished, leaves a residual tension in you. The sense of inferiority that you do not attempt to correct creates in time tensions which have physical, mental, and emotional repercussions. The physical results are tangible enough, but the far-reaching effects, in the shape of the warping of personality, are less tangible. And yet it is these effects which determine your whole attitude toward life, what you will get out of life, your success or failure, the growth and flowering or the distorting and fading of the sum-total of the elements that make up yourself.

Freeing the Personality

Relaxation, as we have pointed out, not only prevents disease and increases your energy, but it enables you to think more clearly and it frees the personality.

A generation growing up under tension never becomes aware of its own potentialities. The child, for instance, who is easily cowed, who is negative in his attitude and depressed instead of optimistic, will react to the proper breathing habits like a cut flower to water.

Tension causes wrong use of the diaphragm and that in turn brings about a negative attitude toward life.

When he is taught to use his diaphragm properly, when he gets the right amount of oxygen and the proper circulation of blood, the child begins to develop a new personality. This can be done even when the tensions arising from fear of shock have so disturbed breathing rhythm that asthma has developed. With his regained sense of aliveness, the child becomes co-operative because he feels an increased ability to do things.

How Tension Affects Personality

1. It fosters a sense of inferiority.
2. It develops a negative mental attitude.
3. It leads to the danger of becoming the Napoleon type, which attempts to compensate for small size by too much drive and too great an expenditure of energy.
4. It inhibits concentration and, through the confusion of nerve impulses, makes a person "all mixed up" mentally so that he finds it difficult to make decisions. This feeling of being all mixed up is becoming an increasing problem not only for the individual but for society at large. The mixed-up person is unhappy, frightened, and easily becomes the victim of any ideology which sounds clear-cut enough to solve his problems without forcing him to do his own thinking.
5. Tension encourages the chronic worrier, because worry grows out of the unfinished problem and the inability to make decisions.
6. Tension leads to delinquency and to crime because the blocked-up energies must find release in some way; this is particularly true of the very young—from early adolescence to coming of age.
7. Tension creates frustrations.
8. Tension can frequently cause personality dislocations, such as are revealed in many cases of homosexuality where the initial problem is a fear of facing the responsibilities inherent in normal sex life. This will be discussed more fully in the chapter dealing with "Sex and Common Sense".

What We Can Do About It

We have got to start with the clear understanding that personality is not a gift from heaven; it is the sum-total of the qualities of your mind, your emotions, and your physical body. It is something that you create, either consciously or unconsciously.

According to industrial analysts, business success depends almost eighty per cent on personality, and only twelve per cent on your trained skills. You spend twelve to sixteen years in acquiring those skills, but how much time and thought have you devoted to developing the other eighty per cent?

Because we know that the mind, the emotions, and the body act and interact upon one another, we know that this is a triple problem that we have to solve.

Let's start with the tangibles— with the physical and muscular tensions of the body.

If you have begun to apply the techniques described in the preceding pages, relaxing one muscle group after the other, learning the art of deep breathing so that you are getting the proper amount of oxygen into your system, regaining muscle flexibility so that your body stays in proper alignment and your carriage is erect, you have discovered a number of benefits :

1. You suffer from less fatigue.

2. You are getting rid of nagging aches and pains.

3. You have released more energy which gives you more self-confidence and more zest for living.

4. With the release of strain and the right posture you have improved your appearance.

5. Beyond all these benefits, you have the feeling of being at peace with yourself that comes with the knowledge that you are tackling your problem, that you are doing something concrete about it.

The Relaxed Person Gets the Job

A young man of twenty-six came to me because he wanted to correct his flat feet. He complained of severe lower back pain that had troubled him for years and for which he could find no cure.

At the moment he was living under a great nervous strain because he had been waiting for several months to be called to an important interview for a government job. For some reason the interview was delayed and delayed.

I used this waiting time to build him up from top to toe. I started by having him lie down and discover his own breathing rhythm, and by so doing begin to find out who and what he was, because the person with a sense of inferiority has lost sight of, and faith in, his own innate personality. I treated his feet, his lower back, his shoulders, and started him on proper breathing habits.

His back pain had got him into the habit of sitting in an awkward position and his flat feet and weak back made him most unimpressive. My first impression was that he was a person without self-confidence.

As soon as he acquired an instinct for proper alignment, his back became stronger; as a consequence, his breathing improved, his back pain disappeared and he began to look better. In his increased confidence, he began to take out girls and to enjoy dancing. He learned to understand what right body function was and then to apply it in his everyday life. For some weeks, of course, he had to be conscious of how he walked, stood and sat, but after that the right body alignment had become a fixed habit and he moved properly without having to be aware of it any longer.

Aside from giving him physical treatments, I rehearsed over and over again with him his imminent interview, so that when the real thing came it would be like an old familiar experience.

He promised to report on the outcome. And he did! What happened when he finally walked into the personnel department was that he felt so relaxed and confident that he was able to show what he really knew, and he made so favourable an impression that he landed a far better job than the one he had hoped to get.

The fear of job hunting is so great in some people that it prevents them from changing jobs, even though they realise that they are not in a place where they are happy or where they can develop to the best of their abilities.

Try to find out for yourself whether this is the reason for your dissatisfaction. If you are afraid of looking for a job, find a friend or relative who will listen and criticise you. Then go through your entrance in the personnel office and the questions and answers that might be expected during your interview. Do this several times, thinking of the questions that you might want to ask the interviewer. If you practise until you can go through the imaginary interview with confidence, you will find that job hunting loses its terrors. If you want to look for another job you can, and you will save yourself the self-reproach you might otherwise have suffered later on when you realised that you were stuck with the wrong job simply because you dared not look for the right one.

Don't be foolhardy, however, and drop your present job and rush out in search of another. It is seldom wise to leave one job until you are certain that something else is ready for you.

The Mental Approach to Personality

While you are a victim of muscular tensions it is almost impossible for you to release your own personality. When you have achieved physical relaxation and acquired the proper feeling of alignment in your body you are ready to approach the problem mentally.

A physical sense of balance helps you to acquire a mental sense of balance. When you have learned to achieve a feeling of quiet in your body, you are better able to achieve a feeling of quiet in your mind. The best use of the mind comes not from driving and tension, but from quiet, which means that you are able to think clearly and to think things through without getting mixed up by the wrong signals.

Worry is a result of conflicting mental ideas and tensions

which result in a person's being unable to make up his mind. The person who worries cannot decide whether to do this or that; he is afraid of what may happen. Suppose that . . . what if . . .

Once you are calm in body and mind, you can look at your problem squarely and decide, "On the basis of all the facts I have, this is the choice I make." When you have made up your mind, the weight of worry tends to fall away. Worry grows overwhelmingly out of indecision, which, in turn, grows out of unreleased tensions.

That's all very well, you say, but I still don't know how to feel relaxed and confident mentally. My answer is: Let's act as though we were not afraid, and see what happens to us.

The next time you go to a party—and don't refuse an invitation because you dread parties and feel like a wallflower when you are a guest at one—don't get yourself in a state of jitters in the first place by worrying about it; and don't key yourself up, thinking you have to be entertaining or die in the attempt. You'll only end with worse nervous tension.

Take a series of long breaths and let every part of your body get completely relaxed. Go in quietly without trying to be the centre of the stage and without trying to hide behind someone else. It isn't the noisy fellow who arouses interest. It is the person who seems to be entirely self-sufficient, controlled, and at ease. He's the one who makes the best impression.

Your own relaxed condition will affect those around you. Because you are relaxed, you will be a keener observer of what is going on and able to talk with interest in someone else. When you can do this, your own self-consciousness will begin to fade away.

CHAPTER FOURTEEN

Sex and Common Sense

PERHAPS nothing has got more attention in the last forty years than the subject of sex. Since Freud, the problem of sex has been under a spotlight. The literature on the subject is mountain high and the Kinsey Report on the sex behaviour of the male has come as a startling reminder of the enormous changes in viewpoint that have taken place in the past half-century. The door that was once closed and marked taboo has now been flung wide open.

And yet, with all this general discussion of the subject, there is still widespread ignorance of sex, fear of sex, lack of normal enjoyment of sex, and a misconception of its place in the life of the average, healthy person.

Advertisements, films, and the jacket illustrations on novels would all suggest that sex is the sole preoccupation of the male and female from adolescence to senescence, the one thought, the only interest, the chief delight—or woe, as the case may be.

This distortion of the subject is as unrealistic as the ostrich attitude of Victorians, who tried to suggest that sex was non-existent.

Actually, when anyone stops to analyse his life, he will see that most of his time and energy is devoted to earning a living, that his thoughts are concerned with a multitude of things from his income tax to his dinner, and that sex, while an important element in his life, does not dominate it. Sex is a normal function of the body like any other and should be regarded in that light.

Fear of Sex

Sex is at the root of the battle of life. The attitude a person takes in regard to sex is a fair index to his general sense of values and his approach to life as a whole. When you approach sex in an attitude of fear, you become seriously handicapped emotionally, create tensions, and throw both your mental and physical life out of true balance.

What are these fears that create so much trouble and frustration?

Adolescents Don't Understand

For the teen-ager, sex fear is perhaps the most common one. The adolescent does not understand what is going on in his own body; he does not know the real meaning of his new feelings, his moods that fluctuate from high expectation to deep melancholy, particularly if he lives in surroundings where there is little sympathy with this difficult period of life. As a result, the child tries to hide his perplexing feelings, largely because he believes that they are bad.

Sex and guilt have been linked in people's minds for so many hundreds of years that they are at the root of an enormous amount of frustration.

How can you suddenly feel so different towards the boy next door? How can you hide those developing breasts that show under your dress? Why do you suddenly discover that your teacher is a marvellous person?

If this adolescent sex anxiety does not, in time, find a normal outlet through marriage, it may be the cause of severe physical tension and mental frustration.

To-day it should be possible for any honest and intelligent adult to find out for himself whether his tensions are the result of such adolescent fears.

The Fear of Pain in Women

This arises almost always from having suffered pain in menstruation. Girls are apt to take menstrual pains for granted and they do not forsee the bad psychological effect of these pains. A girl who suffers every month from menstruation is apt to get a fear complex in regard to this region of her body and she will start her married life with a subconscious fear that often prevents happy sex relations.

A girl had just started her menstruation and these days were a trial for her whole family each month because she suffered such terrible pain that it affected everyone around her. She was a normal, healthy, fifteen-year-old girl and I found nothing wrong. At length I asked her to walk around the room and watched the way she moved and used her body. Then I found the reason for the trouble. She pulled in her stomach as hard as she could.

"Why do you do that?" I asked her.

"Everyone says to do it," she said in surprise. "My dancing teacher and my physical education mistress, and all the beauty columns. Everyone."

I explained to her that this habit was not only harmful to her body as a whole but that it was the cause of the menstrual pains she had been suffering. She was hard to convince. People are always hard to convince when they have a good authority like "Everyone says so".

However, she was eager to be rid of her pain, so she began to change her breathing habits, to keep her diaphragm relaxed, and to learn that the right body alignment would take care of the "stomach in" problem without the harmful pulling.

Ten days later she returned to her home in the Middle West, where her family waited with foreboding for her next period. That was some years ago and the pain has never recurred, as I learned when I again encountered the young woman.

In many cases, proper posture and breathing are not enough to clear up menstrual pains. Frequently, relief can be attained, however, by massage.

You may be startled as you see this picture of the lower leg. Nevertheless, feel the spot marked x on the diagram. If you find sensitiveness, tension or considerable puffiness at this point, start to massage it, even if it is painful. If you massage with a rotating movement, you will notice, after a while—

probably about three minutes—that your legs relax on the inner side and that your ankle joints feel looser.

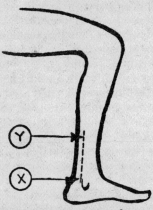

For relief from menstrual cramps, massage between the points shown

The result that comes from massaging from point x to y is often miraculous, causing bad menstrual cramps to disappear in a few mintues. In many cases, the next menstrual period may come without any pain whatever. This massage of the lower leg, combined with correct breathing, will greatly help your menstrual difficulties, except in cases where the cause of the trouble is some internal complication such as a cyst, a tumour, or a prolapse of the uterus. In all these cases, you should get medical attention.

The Fear of Childbirth

Dr. Grantley Dick Read, Fellow of the Royal Society of Medicine and member of the Royal College of Surgeons, has pioneered for many years to convince women that by learning the art of relaxation during pregnancy they can enjoy the birth of their children as a wonderful experience. Childbirth, he tells them, is a natural process. The pain is a result of their own fears and tensions.

He had to fight not only the scepticism of his patients but the whole profession in England. It is only recently, and after having delivered many women in painless childbirth, that his teachings have been understood. At the present time, Yale University is doing interesting and productive research in this field.

Of the possibilities of painless childbirth through relaxation and freedom from fear, I can speak from personal experience. A clever older sister, who was a physician, told me, when I expected my first child, "You must not be afraid. You will enjoy every moment of giving birth if you do not waste your strength when labour starts. Take the first hours easy so that you will have strength for the last minutes."

As a result, the birth of my three children provided me with the greatest moments and the most profound experiences of my life.

Much of the fear of childbirth is a hangover from the days when women had good reason for fear; those days—happily far behind us—when they were exposed to puerperal fever as a result of infection; when they were without X-rays and all the modern safeguards that have made birth so much less hazardous.

Fear of pain and of the risk of giving birth set up tensions which are a major cause of the pain of childbirth.

The pain comes from muscular tension, which is caused by emotional tension in the mind. If the mother begins during the early months of pregnancy to practise relaxation, the muscles which guard the exit to the uterus, and whose tension causes pain, can be so relaxed that the birth is painless.

Relaxation in Pregnancy

The method of relaxation is the same simple one we have been practising throughout this book. Lie down, feeling that the bed, chair, or floor holds your whole weight and that you

185

do not have to support yourself. Take a few deep breaths so that you feel the air stream in and the muscles expanding from the throat clear down to the pelvis. Simple, isn't it?

Whenever a young woman who expects her first baby asks me what method is best for having her babies without pain, I answer, "Want your baby; look forward to its coming with joy; regard the moment of its arrival as the great emotional peak of your life, and relax. If you are without fear and without tension, you will be without pain."

My experience shows that even severely handicapped women can give birth painlessly and enjoy it if they are adequately relaxed.

A girl came to me for help in relaxation. She had been under the care of a famous orthopædist for many years and for eight years had worn a brace because she had a bad curvature of the spine that had thrown her hips and pelvis out of alignment. Her arms were under-developed because of the brace, which prevented her from moving freely, and her breathing was shallow and poor.

After a while the brace was removed and we started the re-education of her body and moving habits. The improvement in her appearance was so striking that compliments flowed in and the improvement these gave her morale stimulated her to carry on her new habits. After five years of treatments once a week, she was married. Shortly before the birth of her first child, she became convinced that childbirth was not to be feared. The doctors told her that if she had a child it must be by Cæsarian operation but she refused so much as an anæsthetic. She wrote to me from the hospital, "I was able to relax while in labour and to enjoy the birth of my daughter as a wonderful, exciting experience. The pains were not too bad and I wish all my friends could have their children this way." A year later she had her second child, still without difficulty.

In her case, relaxation had naturally not straightened a deformed spine, but she had gradually made all her muscles so flexible from head to foot that even those which had suffered

186

from the wrong alignment lost their tension and she never needed to return to a brace.

That childbirth can be experienced as the most natural process in a woman's life is illustrated by the following story of a Polish peasant.

A friend of mine who owned an estate in Poland was interested in teaching the farm workers modern methods of child care and maternity care. In particular, she urged them to consult a physician.

One day she encountered one of her women workers walking home from the field, carrying a basket. The woman, beaming, stopped and asked my friend to look in the basket. It held twins, new born. She explained that she had given birth to the twins in the field and was on her way home. But, she added, proud to show my friend that she understood her teachings, she had stopped on the way to show the children to the doctor!

The Healthy Sex Life

It is disturbing to realise that comparatively few people are able to experience complete sex enjoyment. No healthy sex life is possible without the proper function of the whole person, physically, mentally, and emotionally.

With all the fascinating knowledge we have gained in the field of sex, one very important point has so far been overlooked, and that is the inter-relationship between (1) physical under-development and muscular lack of function and (2) sex behaviour and sex sensations. We have neglected up to now the development of those muscle groups that contribute to the practice of sex.

No period in history has ever given so much open discussion to sex. Indeed, all our life impulses are supposed to be based on sex. Repression and frustration are regarded as underlying causes of most mental and emotional difficulties, but in trying to reveal the complexities of the subconscious we have neglected to improve the sex function and make possible its greatest enjoyment.

Psycho-analysis tries to find the root of maladjusted sex life or unsatisfactory sex relations in hidden fears or complexes, and while the answer may often be found there, the failure to achieve sex satisfaction does not always lie in psychological reasons. Important as the psychological angle is, the physical angle too must be considered. The trouble often lies in physical under-function, to which we are exposed through our living conditions, most damaging of which is unreleased tension. Hundreds of people have been helped to live and enjoy a richer and far more satisfactory sex life simply by releasing the nerve sensations that had been blocked through tension.

Common Sources of Difficulty

Where are the sources of the trouble? Let us start with the under-developed chest and sloping shoulders of the shallow breather. There is a popular saying about the shallow person, "Nothing goes deep". That is apt to be particularly true of the shallow breather, who may become a person with a limited emotional scope. Through the repressions that go with shallow breathing and the shallow chest, a person often does not develop a capacity for deep feeling.

The development of the muscles of the lower back, pelvis and thighs is of far greater importance than the average married man or woman dreams. Certainly it is common sense to pay attention to the normal function of all organs and muscle groups that contribute to the practice of sex.

Look at the flabby buttocks of the average woman. What effect do they have on the practice of sex? Well, more than you think. Curiously enough, with all the pronounced interest in the subject, few people speak out, honestly and frankly, and say that sex can be one of the most pleasurable sensations of life. That when it fails to be pleasurable, it is because in many cases the individual, through muscular and nerve tensions, has blocked or atrophied areas which prevent the sensitive nerves from producing the proper sex sensation.

188

One of these areas is around the hip section. When the buttocks become flabby, this keenness of sensation is blunted. Only when a body functions properly so that no nerves are blocked, either through muscles that are too weak or through being muscle-bound, can the nerve sensation be unimpaired and the practice of sex be enjoyed.

This applies to men, especially those who have over-developed thighs because of playing ball or other sports. Now add to these blocked nerve sensations in the muscles the lack of circulation caused by our sixteen-hour sitting habit and you get still another explanation for many of the male and female sexual difficulties.

The result of these difficulties is repression, because when an impulse is prevented from being carried through, it will result in repression in the brain or frustration. When the sex impulse is thwarted too often, it leaves you with a feeling of depression and dissatisfaction that sets up mental tensions.

Restoring Nerve Sensations

The result achieved by restoring nerve sensations in the legs and lower back has been most gratifying not only in an improved practice of sex but in the blossoming of the whole personality.

A football player came to me for release of tension, and among his other difficulties he explained that he got little satisfaction out of his sex life. I explained that by being muscle-bound in his thighs, he blocked all sensation from his feet to his sex organs.

How was he to improve the condition? By releasing all the muscle groups involved; starting with the lower leg at the Achilles' tendon, at the knee, and the thighs.

We discovered that because of the over-development of the thigh muscles, those in the small of his back and his hips were too weak, and this weakness prevented him from enjoying the sensitiveness that brought the greatest sex gratification.

189

It took only a few weeks before the tensions were released and he was able to resume a satisfactory sex life.

If psychiatrists and psycho-analysts would examine their patients for proper muscular and nerve sensation, many a problem based on sexual difficulties could be solved with less time and financial burden and with the result that the newly developed sex enjoyment would provide more self-confidence and better social relations. My experience with many people in this respect has been most encouraging.

Sex in Middle Age

Many women of middle age become depressed and feel old and unhappy because they lose the sensation of vigour and trimness they had in their youth. They are afraid that their husbands' affection will go to younger women because, even though they succeed in keeping their weight down, their bodies grow flabby.

It is amazing to see how quickly these women change in mind and body when they realise that they can regain this sensation of vigour and youth when they regain proper function of their lower back, buttocks, and thighs. In nearly all these cases the main reason for the feeling of growing old and being without sex attraction is, at the root, shallow breathing. In many cases, the condition is a result of improper body alignment and poor walking habits due to wrong weight distribution as a result of high heels or faulty sitting habits.

The change in mind and body as a result of this physical rejuvenation affects the whole atmosphere of a house. I have seen many mother-daughter relationships, which had been strained because of the hidden resentment of a mother for the blossoming of her daughter, adjusted and restored to their former basis.

The Unmarried Woman

On the other hand, it is the unmarried woman who must

realise that sex plays an exaggerated rôle to-day and that Freudian ideas should not ruin her life by giving her the feeling that she is inferior because she has no children or sexual relations.

It is my own conviction that in at least fifty per cent of these cases, the real problem is not a sex problem so much as it is one of emotional tension. The lack of an emotional outlet is far more disturbing than the lack of sex relations. The need of these women is for someone on whom they can lavish affection, someone on whom they can rely for affection, for a sense of "belonging". They need the emotional security of sharing their problems and their daily lives. They need some way to dispel their loneliness.

They miss having children for whom they can care, whom they can love, and who serve as a link with the next generation.

Some of them try to solve this problem by doing welfare work. Some keep pets and lavish love on them to help them overcome their loneliness. Some find an outlet in teaching the young—that provides a link with the next generation. But these are all substitutes.

I believe that the emotional problem of the unmarried woman deserves far more attention than we have accorded it in the short period of woman's emancipation. The spotlight has been focused almost entirely on sex. This is natural because sex is more dramatic and the woman who breaks through conventions for sex freedom is always a lively subject for discussion and controversy. But it misses the real point, the fact that for at least fifty per cent of the unmarried women it is affection which they need, both in giving and receiving.

What gives the relation of parent and child its deep foundation is the security of having someone who will really stick with you to the end. It is the uncertainty of friendship that is the problem of the unmarried man and woman and I believe that women have the harder lot and suffer more damage through this emotional frustration and repression.

In another way, too, the unmarried woman is penalised for

her state, and that is through the fact that, except in unusual cases, she finds herself more or less isolated socially. The unmarried man is always in demand but the unmarried woman is regarded too often as a social nuisance and tends to be cast aside.

Homosexuality

Since the widespread attention directed to the Kinsey Report, it is no longer possible for us, in any discussion of sex, to overlook blandly the prevalence of homosexuality.

I have observed that in a great number of cases, where the homosexuality is not a result of a glandular imbalance, but a result of seduction in school or college, the victim frequently wants to be freed of this habit and to lead a normal sex life.

Non-glandular homosexuality frequently grows out of hidden fears of responsibility for pregnancy and the resulting consequences of fatherhood. In other cases, it is a hidden fear of being a sexual failure that turns boys from a normal sex life. The fear becomes so deeply rooted that they block themselves completely by tension.

In these cases, learning the art of relaxation will restore self-confidence and release tensions and has, in many cases I have known personally, restored the boy to normal sex life. As we know what fear can do in blocking the normal function of the stomach and heart, it is easy to understand that it can be at the root of sex failure, thus increasing the difficulties, until relaxation has to be practised so that it can be applied under the most trying conditions.

CHAPTER FIFTEEN

The Cure of Insomnia

"OUR SLEEP," declared Alfred Adler, "can be undisturbed only if we are free from tension and sure of the solution of our problems."

In other words, if we release our muscular and mental tensions during the day, we will not be troubled by insomnia at night.

Perhaps you will be encouraged when I tell you that of all the different troubles for which people have come to me for relief, insomnia is the one that responds most quickly and lastingly to applied relaxation.

But there is one basic requirement necessary on your side. *You must really want to get rid of your insomnia.* I have found that many people who complain loudly and constantly about their insomnia, and try all sorts of remedies for it, really love it and do not in their hearts want to be free of it.

In such cases, I have not bothered to teach them the techniques that cure insomnia. I can neither breathe for other people nor relax for them. The only thing I can do in the field of applied relaxation is to make you understand your problem and give you treatments to relieve muscular tension. In many cases, treatments must be repeated again and again, explanations must be read over and over and followed through until you develop in yourself a sensation of your own body alignment, feel the difference between complete and shallow breathing, and learn to change your everyday living habits to avoid sustaining tension or living in the wrong rhythm.

Do You Love Your Insomnia?

One of my first questions, therefore, in cases of insomnia,

after I have heard all the complaints and the list of remedies tried, is an unexpected one.

"Do you really want to get rid of your insomnia or do you love it?"

If the person clings to his insomnia, he realises by my question that I have found him out. He loves his lack of sleep because it gives him something to talk about every day, something to observe in himself, something that excuses him for feeling sorry for himself.

One day a patient asked me to take on the case of her father, who was a longshoreman on the docks. He kept his whole family under tension because of his insomnia. He complained about it, he wanted them to come home early so he would not be disturbed; he gave blow-by-blow descriptions about his nights at breakfast. Everybody suffered from it.

It took time for them to persuade him to come to see me, but finally he appeared and told me all his troubles. We started to relax his breathing and before I had done much he was sound asleep. I let him nap half an hour and then, after having watched him all this time through an open door, I went into the room again. When I entered, his first words were the defiant statement, "I did not sleep one minute." I knew that he would never forgive me for having seen him asleep and I was right. He never came back.

He is one of the hundreds of thousands who love their insomnia, even though they sleep most of the night. It is an emotional outlet, something to be pitied for, something to talk about, and last but not least something by which to dominate those who live with them. These are the ones who cannot be helped because they cling like a burr to their insomnia.

By the way that question—"Do you love your insomnia?" —is answered, it is easy to draw one's conclusions. It is possible to find out which person is really plagued by insomnia and wants to cure it, and which one uses his insomnia as a means of attracting attention and sympathy.

My next step—*your* next step, in this case—is to find out what caused your insomnia and why it started in the first place.

It may have started at a time when you were ill and were kept awake by pain. Habit is insidious and a powerful thing. If you became accustomed to waking up at a certain hour because pain usually started at that time, you may simply have continued to do so, even when the reason for it was past. In these cases, the pupil will learn how to relax and not lie tense, waiting for the pain which no longer exists. Once he understands that the pain has formed a muscular and mental habit, he is able to eliminate it.

Many people have a tendency to sleep for some hours and then to awaken around two or three in the morning. They are relieved of their first fatigue and so they feel fine. Now, in the stillness of the night and in privacy, they start to indulge in thinking or to let their fantasy race free. They make plans for the future, or think of unhappy situations in which they find themselves, their thoughts revolving endlessly like a squirrel in a cage. If this night thinking is allowed to become a habit, it may easily be the root of real insomnia, and therefore it must be eliminated.

Night Thinking

As a rule, night thinking causes more harm than good—though there are exceptions, as we shall see later on.

In general, perspective seems to be lost at night. Fears grow to mountains and hopes to towers. We have all experienced the unreliability of the ideas we get and the conclusions we arrive at and the decisions we make in the night. In the daylight these hopes and fears have to stand the cold glare of reality and we realise how much we have exaggerated and distorted values during the night.

But the true insomnia lover waits—though often unconsciously—for these hours of the night when he can indulge, undisturbed, in thoughts and fantasies. Therefore, he awakens around two or three o'clock, eager and ready to take up his dreams, his substitutes for satisfying living.

People of this type are apt to be completely exhausted in the morning, because the constant thinking wears them out, just as does any other type of overwork or orgy. The victim, generally one of those who are disappointed in love or friendship, or who feel they are failures in their work, or who lack self-confidence and a sense of security in dealing with others, uses these night hours to re-live situations in which he has failed, belatedly tackling them with courage and making the bold answers he would like to have made at the time. He is courageous only with shadows.

A middle-aged woman came to me because she suffered from insomnia. She had gone through a period of great stress, acute unhappiness, and real despair.

In her case, the insomnia had become a habit fixed for years, because the nights had been the only time when she could let down the screen behind which she had made it a practice to live. People who met her always found her cheerful and apparently interested. She had waited, year in and year out, for the moment when she went to bed and could be herself and face her disappointment and difficulties.

Instead of looking back, I taught her to look forward. We started relaxing with the goal of making her fit, so that she could study and prepare herself for a new career.

She stopped using her night hours as a time to think about her misery and looked forward to sleeping because the next day brought so much interest that she could keep up only by being rested so that she would be able to concentrate.

If this group of wilful insomnia seekers were to accept the unwelcome fact that they are not victims of sleeplessness; that, instead, they are deliberately keeping themselves awake so that, in their imaginations, they can compensate for their shortcomings during the day, they would reach the next step. They would realise that this sort of "night life" gets them nowhere. Only by building up more strength and vitality will they be able to overcome their difficulties. If they keep on as they are going, they simply make themselves more and more exhausted and less able to cope with the situation. Once they really want to sleep, they will be able to do so—and by so doing they will be in far better shape to get their satisfaction out of reality rather than shadows.

In these cases, the person must learn to be strict with himself. When he wakes up in the night, he must resist the temptation to start thinking. He must have the courage to turn on his side, start deep, relaxed breathing, and wish ardently to go back to sleep.

Pleasant Insomnia

Every one of us has experienced times when he could not sleep; for instance, when he had to make a really far-reaching decision.

At such times, you will wake up about three o'clock in the morning and start to think things over. To your surprise you will be able to see the pros and cons clearly and arrive at your decision. These are also the hours known to all people who have creative gifts; hours when they awaken and enjoy the surprise of their own intuition or vision.

If these times come—they sometimes last for weeks and sometimes only for a short time—you must realise that they should not be allowed to get out of control and become a habit. When your decision has been made, self-control should tell you that it is no longer necessary for you to awaken at this hour and lose your sleep. The waking period was a necessary step for growth and development, but it has served its purpose.

I know a famous surgeon who told me, "Whenever, in doubtful cases, I have to make the far-reaching decision of whether or not to operate, I think it through carefully before I go to bed. Then I can be sure that I will awaken about three o'clock and know clearly what I should do. It is the first thought in my mind when I awaken and I go back to sleep immediately. Whenever I stick to this decision, I am right;

whenever I have let myself be influenced by conferences with colleagues to make a different decision, I have regretted it.''

Business men and many other professional people have told me of the same experience.

There is another type of pleasant insomnia—times when you lie awake for several hours for no particular reason. Of course, if you want to get excited about the situation, the insomnia won't be pleasant. But if you relax and enjoy the quietness of the night, and the comfort of having a bed and a roof and are grateful for the security you enjoy, these hours will be restful. They will do you as much good as though you were sound asleep.

This sort of sleeplessness is so pleasant for a short time that it does not occur to you to mention it as sleeplessness to yourself because you feel refreshed in the morning. Usually this sort of sleeplessness is of short duration and, because it does not disturb you, it vanishes completely after several days.

What Causes Insomnia?

Before we try to put a stop to your habit of insomnia, let's look at the various things that keep you awake.

With advancing age, people need fewer hours of sleep, *but they need more rest.* Because they are accustomed to spending a certain number of hours in bed, and the members of the household are getting the usual number of hours of sleep, they are apt to be distressed by their own sleeplessness and to feel that something is wrong.

For the elderly, the only sensible solution is to accept the fact that they sleep less because they need less sleep. Instead of worrying about it or tossing fretfully, why not turn on the light and read for a while, or get up at an earlier hour than the rest of the household, thus adding more pleasant hours to the day instead of more restless hours to the night? The over-whelming number of these cases compensate for broken nights by frequent dozing and cat naps during the day.

Often, it is small problems that prevent people from making this simple adjustment. "I can't start the morning without a cup of coffee," someone says fretfully. "I'll just lie in bed and wait until someone gets up and prepares it." Why not have a Thermos bottle of coffee prepared at night so that it is ready for you in the morning? Then you will start your early morning pleasantly, have the coffee you need, and be willing to wait patiently until others are stirring.

Illness

Nearly every illness, certainly any illness accompanied by pain, is likely to cause temporary insomnia because of physical discomfort. Any case of interrupted breathing, such as the common cold, hay fever, or asthma, produces, is apt to cause a certain amount of insomnia. The cure for this type of insomnia obviously depends on clearing up the physical condition.

Digestive upsets, indigestion, constipation, and the like are frequent offenders in causing insomnia, and here too, once you trace the cause, the remedy is obvious.

Hardening of the arteries, in those over middle age, frequently leads to insomnia. This complaint affects nervous people far more severely than it does those who are relaxed; and it is more evident in the case of those who indulge heavily in alcohol. Therefore, the knowledge that the elasticity of the blood vessels is impaired need not make you feel the condition is hopeless if you are willing to retrain yourself in the art of relaxation.

Chronic diseases are a serious problem in insomnia, because some chronic diseases, such as arthritis, or neuritis, tend to increase in painfulness at night. In these cases, where the patient expects his pain because he knows from experience that he is going to suffer at night, learning to relax can work miracles if the patient really wants to sleep and has not become so dependent on sedatives that he has lost the energy to try and help himself.

If he will concentrate on relaxation through breathing it will take his mind off the expectation of his pain and frequently bring sleep before the pain starts, the onset of pain sometimes being due to mental and emotional causes that make him tense.

An over-active thyroid also leads to high nervous tension and causes acute wakefulness, but this is a case for your doctor to treat.

Fatigue

It is a well-known fact that the more tired you are the more difficult it is for you to rest. That is why we keep stressing the importance of taking it easy, of recuperating as you go along, of learning how to budget your energy.

If you are over-tired, you are so keyed up that you fail to relax the muscle groups and therefore you go to bed in a state of tension. It is interesting to observe that the restless sleeper, the person who tosses and twists, who turns his pillow and thumps it, who pulls up the blankets and tosses them off again, who moves his head in an increasing endeavour to find a more comfortable spot, is most apt to be a person who lives in the same restless way during his daytime hours. He is the one who is constantly getting up to shut or open the window, who shifts his position over and over again in his chair, who cannot seem to be comfortable.

In the daytime, all these restless movements increase his fatigue; in the night, they increase his wakefulness. Each time he moves he gets wider awake.

In other words, this is a person who is basically dissatisfied. He has not found what he wants. He is constantly and restlessly on the search for it. During the day he is trying tirelessly to attain something he has not got; at night he is seeking for an unattainable sort of comfort before he will try to sleep. But sleep will not come after he has attained this comfort; sleep must come first and the comfort will come with it.

If this restless person is you, you must realise first that you are keeping yourself awake by your own actions; second, that you must train yourself to relax, then to lie still; third, and most difficult, of course, you must think through what it is you are after and then go after it during the day by a clear-cut plan. Constant hopping around in perpetual motion wears you out without taking you a step closer to your goal.

Anxiety

This brings us back to the quotation from Alfred Adler's *What Life Should Mean to You,** with which we opened this chapter: "Our sleep can be undisturbed only if we are free from tension and sure of the solution of our problems."

The unsolved problem, the uncompleted job, the unmade decision, all leave residual tensions. Every night thousands of people toss on their beds, staring blindly into the darkness, kept awake not because they are trying to solve their problem but simply because they have not solved it. The thing nags at them, nibbles at the edge of their consciousness even when they seem to be thinking about something else, it goads at them.

There is no such thing as running away from the unsolved problem. You can set out for a deserted island but your problem will be waiting on the shore to greet you. You can pretend to yourself that it does not exist and it will be like the splinter that you did not bother to remove. It will fester under the skin until it comes out. The only problem you are through with is the one you have faced. That one does not keep you awake at night.

Fear of Insomnia

It is a curious thing that a chief factor in keeping us awake at night is the fear that we won't go to sleep. A few sleepless nights seem to engender fear and then the fear keeps us awake. "I won't be able to sleep," you tell yourself as you get into

* Allen & Unwin Ltd.

bed. "I'll toss around all night and I'll be all worn out in the morning. Limp as a rag. And I'll look awful too. My mind won't be clear enough to handle my work."

By this time you have begun to work yourself into a fine state of jitters. You've told yourself so often that you can't sleep that you believe it. You lie awake to watch yourself lie awake. You grow more and more tense. Your breathing rhythm is thrown out of balance.

The Little Things Again

In many cases of insomnia it has been possible to restore normal sleep as soon as we got to the root of the trouble. The things that were causing tension and sleeplessness were frequently trivial in themselves. In one case, for instance, the person, who was an unusually orderly person, was kept awake by irritation over the untidiness of the bedroom; in other cases it has been an uncomfortable bed, or a room that was too hot or too cold. Sometimes this discomfort is real, more often it is imaginary.

There is a story I heard long ago of two travellers who had to share a room in an over-crowded inn. One man could sleep only with a window open, the other only if it were closed. After a heated argument, the fresh-air addict had his way and flung open the casement window. He slept happily while the other man tossed all night. In the morning, they learned that what they had taken in the dark for a casement window was a cupboard door.

Some people find that it helps them to go to sleep if they read in bed; others find that this makes them more wakeful.

You may have acquired the habit of eating your chief meal too late in the evening, and if circumstances make it impossible for you to take a short leisurely walk in quiet surroundings before going to bed, you probably sit the short time after your meal with little or no movement, so when you go to bed your over-loaded stomach is the cause of your tossing around.

If this is the case with you, revise your schedule so that you will dine earlier and have more time in which to digest your meal before going to bed. If you are accustomed to eating early, you may be ready for a light snack before you go to bed, but that has a calming rather than an upsetting effect. I mean a glass of milk, an apple, or some biscuits. Not lobster sandwiches. But be careful with sweets at a late hour. They have a disastrous effect on sleep.

A temporary reason for interrupted sleep at night may be sudden pain, a toothache, intestinal mix-up, or an injury. But you will realise that these temporary disturbances will vanish when the cause has been taken care of.

Insecurity, Enemy of Sleep

If the cause of your insomnia is not physical you will find that the root is always fear. But the fear may be so disguised that you do not realise it.

Modern child psychology stresses the point of giving children a feeling of security, of belonging somewhere, as the most important source of healthy development. We all know how good it feels to go to bed with the comforting sensation of being at home, secure and protected.

Those of us—and there are hundreds of millions of us to-day —who have known what it was, because of war and political persecution, to lose this feeling of belonging somewhere and being secure, know that it sometimes takes months to be able to regain the sense of security, although the hours of danger are past. But we do not need to be in danger of our life to lose sleep. Small things can have the same effect if we allow them to overcome us with hidden anxieties.

There is the examination that lies ahead for the school or college pupil. In the dark of the night you think of all the classes you missed, of the pages you skipped, of the things you do not know. They grow to mountains so that you forget how much work you really did and how much knowledge you have actually acquired.

If you have learned to relax, you can handle this situation

without difficulty. You tell yourself firmly, "I will need my strength and concentration to-morrow. Therefore, the only thing to do is to stop this nonsense. I am going to yawn because that makes me sleepy, then I will sleep and do my best to-morrow."

This is a question of self-education, of deliberately breaking into your worries to concentrate on yawning and relaxing.

Perhaps you have to face a decision which is important for your own life or that of a member of your family. Perhaps you will drop off to sleep without difficulty because you are worn out, but in the middle of the night you will wake up and begin to worry.

If your worry makes you afraid, force yourself to breathe deeply. Fear checks your breathing and the longer you hold your breath the more tense you become.

A deep breath helps break every fear spell! If you read this sentence again and again, you will be safe for life from most fear tensions because you will be able to help yourself.

Too Tired to Sleep

In studying your insomnia, find out whether you are too tired when you go to bed. This exhaustion may mean that you are tense and unable to let go. That is one of the reasons we are trying to show you how to *avoid* getting exhausted. In case of real exhaustion, one night of sleep and rest is not enough to restore your health balance.

People understand that if they spend too much money it will take time to get their bank account balanced, and that they will have to put in more money than they need for their usual expenses to make up the deficit. But, in regard to exhaustion and health, few realise this same fundamental truth. One night is not enough to restore you if you went to bed late for a whole week or if you have lived under great strain. You will need several nights of more sleep to balance your exhaustion. You cannot go on living like a spendthrift when it comes to your health fortune.

Find out your most agreeable sleeping conditions. Some like a warm cover, some need little warmth. Some sleep better with an open window, some need it closed. Some sleep better with the blinds down in a dark room, others prefer no blinds. Some like a hard mattress and others prefer it soft. No single advertised sleep inducer will help everybody.

What About Sleeping Pills?

That depends. If a person has been accustomed to taking sedatives for a long time, it may be wrong to urge him to cut them out completely because that might upset him. In nearly all cases, the progressive ability to relax and enjoy better sleep makes the use of sedatives unnecessary. As soon as the victim of insomnia feels that they are unnecessary to help him sleep, they become unimportant in his mind and he begins to forget to take them. Once he has forgotten, the habit is broken and the fixed idea—"I cannot sleep without my pills"—is interrupted.

On the other hand, I find a light sedative helpful for a short time if the person is exposed to great nervous strain and lack of sleep would expose him to great tension.

The night before an examination or an important meeting, a sedative is frequently helpful. In this case, it does not matter whether the person takes a sugar pill. The fact that he has taken something assures him that sleep will come and that he will feel rested the next morning. It is a psychological help in a difficult moment and there is no risk of forming a habit.

The dangers of powerful, habit-forming sleeping pills are obvious. To begin with, the person who takes them finds it most difficult to learn to relax and sleep without their help. In the second place, it is frequently necessary to increase the dose in order to continue to get the same benefit from them. In time, they have a bad effect on both mind and body.

The solution of insomnia is not drugs but common-sense techniques that will produce normal, healthy sleep.

In times when people lived in accordance with the seasons of the year, rising early in summer, and sleeping long in winter, they also respected a most important time of the day—the hour that brings a natural demand for rest and calming down. I mean the hour of dusk.

Up to a hundred years ago, twilight was the end of the working day, for the farmer as well as for the artisan. They had to follow daylight, because it was too expensive to use candles or oil lamps.

With the invention of gas and electric light, people began to ignore the rising and setting of the sun, and to make a profound change in the rhythm of their living habits. Twilight became a time when the lights were switched on and activities continued without pause.

But what happened in those earlier days when twilight fell? Gradually, all the members of a household stopped work and gathered in one place—usually in the kitchen. Those of you who live in the country know that instinctively people fall into a quiet and peaceful mood at dusk. Voices are lower, conversation gradually stops. Men come home from the fields. The quietness that settles over the earth influences your movements. Everything slows down. This is the time when mothers gather their children around them and tell them stories.

By living according to the rhythm of the day, people calm down early in the evening. Their rhythm becomes slow and relaxed, their nerves and minds are at ease, and by the time they go to bed it is easy to sleep.

But in the city we live not in accordance with the natural rhythm of the seasons or the change from daylight to dark, but by an artificial rhythm which completely ignores the twilight hour, and the wonderful quietness which nature brings. Aside from being deprived of this slowing-down time, we are subjected to a constant impact of outside impressions. In an overwhelming number of cases, there is little real quiet in the home. There is too little space; there are too many people; it is almost impossible to be alone so that you can find the quiet you need. In your living-room there is probably either a radio or a television screen assailing your ears or your eyes.

To try to fall into a restful sleep immediately after all these disturbances is naturally more difficult than it is for the country man, whose nerves have been relaxed since twilight, to fall asleep.

In all cases, I try to induce the sufferer to help himself. He has to report on the methods he finds best for him because here, as in so many ailments, people tend to rely on the help of a person who prescribes a drug or gives some other form of treatment, and they rarely resort to their own initiative to restore their own health.

How relaxation can help in all these cases was indicated by research done in the air force with a group of cadets. They were watched at night, their restlessness and constant turning was checked. Then they were taught relaxation techniques. On checking their night habits again, the physicians discovered that their restlessness and shifting had been reduced by fifty per cent!

My experience has proved that men who carry great responsibilities are especially likely to be victims of insomnia. In nearly all these cases the responsibility overpowers the person. It may be financial responsibility. Many bankers are insomnia victims. It may be the responsibility for other people whose jobs depend on the decisions made by one man.

Childhood Memories

In all these cases, I found a simple remedy of the utmost value. After teaching the basic techniques of applied relaxation, I ask these men to lie down in their most comfortable sleeping position and to forget their job, concentrating on the voice and the sensation of the comforting hand that put them to bed when they were small boys of three or four. Sometimes it was the mother, sometimes a grandmother or a nurse, but whoever it was, she brought a feeling of security. As the man begins to recall that sensation, subconsciously he starts to relax and after some moments he will sleep. This remembrance of childhood experiences, of being put to bed with a kind word, a good-night, and a light pat on the head, works wonders in over-burdened executives. Many have made it a habit to recapture these childhood memories and told me that it helped them to overcome insomnia.

A young banker who suffered for years from insomnia confessed that he lay stiff and tense as a rod and that he felt exhausted in the morning. As soon as he learned what tension did, not only to his body but also to his mind, he was cured.

How to Sleep

This is a problem that requires both physical and mental relaxation. Lie down in a comfortable position.

As you lie there, take an inventory of yourself. Your jaw should be relaxed from yawning, your eyes are closed, your forehead and facial muscles are relaxed without frowning, the tip of your tongue rests behind your lower teeth.

Now take a few deep breaths. Exhale forcibly with a shhing sound that forces down the diaphragm. Your arms are relaxed; there is no tension in feet or legs. If your legs feel tense, do the leg stretch (page 98), remembering to start the pull at the heel.

It is understood, of course, that you have taken no problems to bed with you for solution, and that you are not afraid that you will not sleep. Suppose you don't? If you have sense enough to lie still, you will get almost the same amount of rest and no harm will be done, so what frightens you?

Don't let your thoughts control you—you control them. Give your mind a rhythmic picture—waves washing up over the sand as the tide comes in; one wave and another and another; as far out as you can see, an unending succession of waves rolling in and over the sand.

Now let the rhythm slow down and stop. There is nothing

in your mind at all. Resist the temptation to shift your position. You won't be more comfortable in the next one. Each movement helps to keep you awake. Shut your mind to the thoughts that come in. Your sagging jaw and the tongue touching your lower teeth help to give you a feeling of mental emptiness.

You won't master this technique the first night or the second. The way you sleep is a result of the way you have lived your day. If you have mastered the art of relaxation *as you went along,* so that you are not over-tired; if you have released your energy instead of storing it up in tension; if you have faced your problems and come to a decision about them (remember that worry is simply a sign you haven't made up your mind); if you have solved your emotional problems instead of waiting for bedtime to relive them on a happier plane; you will not be troubled with insomnia. When you have learned to live on twenty-four hours a day—and we'll discuss that in a later chapter—you will learn how to sleep.

"Yes, but——" you begin.

And I answer roundly, "Yes, you can."

Out in the West a road rises from flat country and starts a steep, precipitous, dangerous curve. And where the road curves there is a sign reading, "Yes, you can. Millions before you have done it."

CHAPTER SIXTEEN

How to Use Hobbies

A HOBBY is any activity that you engage in for the sheer joy of doing it, a spare time occupation that has significance and meaning for you. Ideally, of course, that is not only what your job or profession should be, it is what your whole life should be. But since most of us must be content with the next best thing, let's make our hobby so absorbing and satisfactory that it provides a compensation for the hours of drudgery.

In this new, enriched life that we are planning for ourselves, the choice of a hobby becomes of paramount importance, because it must not only give you something to look forward to with anticipation and delight, not only provide you with mental and emotional satisfaction, but—if you are wise—it will supplement your daily activities by providing an outlet for your unused energies.

The average sedentary worker uses his mind to a far greater extent than he uses his hands. He does not discharge as much energy as he should through his muscles and accordingly—yes, you guessed it!—stores it up in the form of tension. If possible, then, your hobby should provide you— if you are a sedentary worker—with some sort of physical outlet. But there is another point to be considered. If you come home from work and paint the back steps, you are getting physical exercise, but it does not constitute a hobby unless you enjoy painting the back steps. A hobby, remember, is something you like to do, something you can hardly wait to get at, something that is fun.

Walking as a Hobby

Let's start with the simplest of all physical activities, and one that is available to everyone at no cost—taking long walks out of doors.

This is one of the best means of releasing tension. Our grandfathers knew that a walk through the woods or along a country road not only refreshed them but that it was also a good way of thinking things over before a decision was made, a help in clarifying ideas and getting new impressions.

The soothing effect of an outdoor walk prevents or calms down many a misunderstanding in marriage and between friends.

Living with nature gives you a sense of proportion. A tree that has stood for 150 years, one of those beautiful maples that dominate so many farmhouses in the eastern states, has a soothing influence on everyone who lives near it. The tree is a silent reminder of the shortness of your life. When you sit under such a tree for a while, your anger will begin to dissolve and your perspective will change as you grow quieter. Why? Because your breathing is influenced and grows slower and deeper, thus relaxing your tense nerves. These big trees give off so much oxygen that you are invigorated as well as relaxed. With the relaxation, your emotions get under control, your brain gets perspective, and your attitude is changed towards your problem.

Remember in walking, however, that cement pavements tire the feet and make them hot and strained, and tired feet mean tired bodies and hence tired nerves. If you are to get real advantage from your walking, you must walk on dirt roads. You will find these in near-by parks if it is impossible to get out into the country.

Too much trouble? Not if it is fun. If you are really going to make walking a hobby, there are dozens of ways in which you can constantly renew its interest. One young couple took a street map of their city and set out, wearing proper shoes, to cover every foot of it by walking, marking the map in coloured chalk as they completed each street. It was so much fun that they have used their summer vacations ever since to cover other cities in the same way.

You can make a list of the historical shrines and other points of interest in and near your city, and make these your goal. It is always surprising to discover how little people know about their own communities, outside of their own immediate circles.

Combining Walking With Other Hobbies

You can use your walking tours for botanical studies or the study of birds. There are a multitude of books for beginners in these various fields that will serve as a guide and you will not only have helpful exercise but you will acquire a fascinating new interest which you can continue to follow up at home through books at times when it is impossible to go walking. Once you acquire a real love for walking, however, you will discover that no weather seems too severe to tempt you out for exercise and the sheer joy of walking.

Or you might find an old camera around the house and decide to combine your walking trips with photography. With mind and eyes alert in search of interesting subjects for pictures, the pleasure of your walk will be doubled.

In fact, if you are to get any benefit out of any hobby, you must approach it with zest. Its whole purpose is to make you happy. Don't set out grimly to walk for your health. Walking is not a penance. It is a privilege. Ask anyone who is lame. I know of no more depressing sight than to stroll around the reservoir in New York City's Central Park on a Sunday morning and look at the faces of the people marching around it. Each of them wears a "do or die" expression; they plod around as though they were on a treadmill. They might as well wear a placard, "I've been told to walk for my health and I'll do it if it kills me".

If you want to add an element of challenge to walking, get a pedometer which will tell you how far you have gone. But don't set yourself a goal and then "walk if it kills you". Either it's fun or there's no sense in it. Remember you are going to walk relaxed, with your body in proper alignment, feeling the air stream past your body, your legs swinging from the hips. Walk down the street as though you owned it.

Swimming Gives Strength and Fun

Perhaps you could get in a swim once a week all the year round. This is an inexpensive sport, available in almost every community. It develops all the muscle groups evenly and improves your breathing habits. If you have failed to swim well in the past, try it again. In nearly all cases where swimming attempts were unsuccessful, the reason for the failure was wrong breathing habits. If you have begun to practise proper breathing, you will find that it is much easier for you now and swimming may become your favourite sport. There is another advantage too. Age is no drawback. *But don't go in for competitions if you are over twenty-five.* That advice applies to all the hobbies mentioned in this chapter. Competition means strain and our goal is relaxation. You don't need to be a channel swimmer. Take it easy and enjoy the floating.

Folk Dancing

If walking and swimming seem dull to you and you want a lot of fun along with your exercise and want to share it with someone else, what about joining a folk-dancing group? This is fun for the whole family and an ideal form of relaxation. Find out whether some of your friends and neighbours would like to join.

What about space? If none of the group has a room large enough, the landlord of your flats—if you live in a block of flats—might find a room in the basement that you can fix up for the benefit of all the tenants. You won't need a trained person to call the dances as you can get records which have been made for this purpose—though it is more fun to have one of the group take over this job as soon as you have learned the routines.

You might like to start a group in which all ages join, or

you might start a folk-dancing group for the children and grow so enthusiastic that you start your own group.

Folk dancing not only enables you to get a lot of physical exercise and to release energies in an enjoyable way but it enables you to follow your own inborn rhythm, which is always an advantage.

Ballroom Dancing

If folk dancing does not appeal to you, why not make a regular habit of ballroom dancing? There are a number of commercial classes but they don't serve the same purpose as home parties with the rugs rolled up and the radio or a gramophone providing the music. If the accent is put on having fun instead of on expense for refreshments and elaborate details of entertaining, which only leaves you tired, you will get a lot out of this.

The point is to keep it informal. Ask your friends and neighbours to come in and join you. It is a fine way for unmarried people to get acquainted. And before long you will find yourself looking forward to the dance as the bright spot of the whole week. Dancing can be enjoyed without age limit. Movement to music relaxes you, increases your flexibility, and puts you mentally at ease.

And there is no question that it makes the week brighter and puts a glow on every day when you have something to look forward to, something that you know is going to be fun. Half the general depression and gloomy spirits you see around you are a result of feeling that life is savourless, and there's nothing ahead, no objective. Setting a goal for the end of the week will help to relieve the tedium of the days in between and do you a lot of good.

Skating

If you are on the look-out for more strenuous exercise, make a hobby of ice skating or roller skating. Both of them are fine for you. Suppose you do take a few spills. You aren't trying to be Sonja Henie; you just want a good work-out and the feeling of swift motion.

Try it for fun and you'll be surprised to see how you limber up and how your muscular co-ordination improves. The first time you'll probably be black and blue and feel disgusted with yourself. Well, don't forget that happened to everyone the first time. Promise yourself that you will give it a fair trial—say, three or four times—before deciding that it is not for you. It will take your body a little time to learn weight shifting and to meet the new muscular demands made on it. But your muscles can do it as well as those of the other people you watch enviously. They can do whatever you give them a fair chance to do.

Remember, when you start on a strenuous hobby, that the idea is not to become a champion. The idea is to become a relaxed and therefore a complete person. There is no merit in tiring yourself out. Rest when you find that you are getting tired. The sport is your toy; it is not to become your master.

Music

Too much of contemporary interest in the arts as a form of expression appears in passive listening. "Spectator sports". That's a terrible phrase. Being a spectator does nothing for you. It is participation that counts. Watching a game gives you no exercise. Listening to music does not help you to express yourself creatively. Every man and woman was born with creative qualities that struggle for expression and too often are given no outlet at all.

Perhaps you would like to join a singing group instead of listening to the radio. Singing is one of the most stimulating hobbies you can take up. The increased breathing relaxes and invigorates your body while the melody and rhythm stimulate your mind. There is an old saying that people who sing together never quarrel with each other, and this has proved true in my own experience.

Did you play the piano as a child? Why not take it up again? I don't mean that you should start practising for hours a day and try to compete with Horowitz. But you will be able to accompany your children at their violin practice or when they are singing and get an immense amount of personal satisfaction through the self-expression this affords.

Nothing brings more pleasure and—if you will forgive me— harmony to a family than making music together. It is the best way of teaching music appreciation and your children will remember these hours of family music all their lives.

Nothing attracts people like music. Before long you will find yourself surrounded by other music-loving friends and your musical Sunday afternoons in the winter months will be a high point in your family life. Perhaps you will prepare Christmas and Easter music which friends and relatives will enjoy hearing and participating in. Home music often brings deeper satisfaction than expensive concerts because you have the satisfaction of making it yourself.

If you haven't a piano or a violin or a 'cello, perhaps you have a guitar or a banjo or a ukulele. There should be some instrument for making music, for this earliest of the arts is a fundamental need in man's nature. He may be colour blind and he may be too undisciplined or mentally incurious to read, but rhythm is in his own nature, in his heart-beat, his breathing, his waking and sleeping, in the core of his personality.

Making Things

It becomes more and more apparent that the man or woman who works with his hands is less apt to become neurotic and dissatisfied with his life than the one who does brain work to the exclusion of the use of his hands. There is infinite satisfaction in the use of the hands, in seeing a concrete object that one has made. A well-known sculptress remarked on the effect on her pupils of working with moist clay, creating a portrait by the use of their hands. Veterans suffering with battle fatigue, women struggling with neuroses, retired elderly men who felt that they had finished their active lives, all became absorbed in the work of creation and as the work progressed, their mental and nervous troubles dropped away.

Your hands were made for use. There is no superiority in having an educated brain and illiterate hands. Put them to work. Teach them to do things. It will give you a feeling of independence and self-reliance to know that you can use your hands for practical purposes. And their use will make you a better-rounded person, for your hands were given you to carry out the ideas in your brain.

If you are a mechanically minded person, how about a hobby room for carpentry or radio building? I see you smile. In my three-room flat, there is no space for a hobby room. Imagine the clutter of tools on the living-room floor and the sound of the hammer after the baby goes to sleep.

But what about the spare room in the basement that might have been used for folk dancing? Talk it over with the other tenants. Perhaps they too would like to use this room for purposes of their own. Talk it over with them and then approach your landlord together. If you offer to fix it up yourself, he may be willing to allow you its use. Then fix it up as a workshop which other tenants can use for their folk dancing or their own particular hobbies on other evenings or at times that won't disturb your own activities.

This unused basement room might become a source of health and happiness for many of you. You might even build some furniture for your wife or a bookcase for your son or a lamp for your daughter or a radio for yourself.

Making things is one of the greatest, direct sources of satisfaction, because it is accompanied by a sense of accomplishment. "See, I did this with my own hands."

Albert Schweitzer, who has done such magnificent pioneer work in Africa, wrote in his *More from the Primeval Forest* of the disastrous effects that come from attempting to skip the normal steps of civilisation and impose our contemporary

Western civilisation on the blacks of Africa before they have taken the intermediate steps.

"How true it is, after all," he wrote, "that civilisation does not begin with reading and writing but with manual labour. Because we have no manual workers here, real progress is impossible. The natives learn to read and write without learning at the same time to use their hands. With these accomplishments they obtain posts as salesmen and clerks, and sit about in white suits. But manual work is despised.

"Had I any say in the matter, no black man would be allowed to read and write without being apprenticed to some trade. No training of the intellect without simultaneous training of the hands! Only so can there be a sound basis for further advance. How ridiculous it seems to me to read that Africa is being opened up to civilisation because a railway has been built to this place, a motor-car has got through to that, and an air service is being established between two other localities. This does not mean any real gain. 'How far are the natives becoming efficient men?' That is the one thing that matters. . . . All other things have meaning only when this foundation has been well and truly laid. . . ." *

Surely it is unnecessary to say that the reference to "black men" was made only as it applied to a particular stage of civilisation under particular circumstances. The point so tellingly made applies with equal force to all men everywhere. The use of the hands is a vital stage in our development as complete human beings. The helpless woman is as antiquated as the dodo. The person, man or woman, who can use his hands efficiently is a more useful and a better-rounded person.

Gardening

A delightful way of combining the use of the hands with the benefits of the out-of-doors is gardening. Perhaps you have friends in the country who would appreciate your help over

*On the Edge of the Primeval Forest and More From the Primeval Forest by Albert Schweitzer. A. & C. Black Ltd.

week-ends, or you might be able to lease an empty plot of ground and start a small garden of your own. If an outdoor garden is impracticable you can start to cultivate some plants in your home.

If the apartment has no sun for blooming plants, get some evergreens. You will be delighted to see how they improve your home and what joy and satisfaction you get out of their care. The appearance of each new leaf is a surprise to be watched. After a while you will learn to understand the needs of the more difficult plants, and water and place them accordingly. Perhaps some day you will be inspired, as a result of tending your plants, to live in a suburb or on a farm where you can enjoy trees and flowers. A few green plants have performed miracles in arousing a love of the out-of-doors in city people.

Hobbies for the Housewife

So far, there has been no mention of the housewife in this chapter on hobbies. In general, the housewife's duties keep her tied to her home, her children, her housework, shopping and meals. The chief complaint of the housewife is that she is always doing the same thing all over again.

For the housewife, therefore, the basic need is for an outside interest among new faces. The idea of women's clubs is a sound one because it meets a pressing need in the housewife's life. Here again it doesn't matter what kind of club—whether bridge or politics, gardening or sports, cultural or sewing for the church. The important thing is that she should have an active interest in a group outside her home where she will be meeting other people. But most important is the fact that she must be interested in it and look forward to it with pleasure.

Choosing Your Hobby

The chief points to bear in mind in selecting your hobby are:

1. It must be something you like doing. Don't choose it because someone else likes it or because it is in fashion or

because you think it is "good for you". It must have significance and meaning for you; it must be something you look forward to doing and do with enthusiasm.

2. Remember that the purpose of the hobby is to increase your happiness and your well-being. Don't work so hard at it that you are all worn out. Even if it is a strenuous form of physical exercise, approach it when you are relaxed and stop to rest when you feel fatigue.

3. Use your ingenuity to find new ways to keep it fresh and interesting. Vary your routines so that it never becomes deadening or automatic.

4. The more of yourself you put into your hobby, the more you will take out in the satisfactions of accomplishment, of self-expression, of the development of your creative instincts, and in just plain joy.

5. Most of the suggestions made above were designed for the sedentary worker. For the person whose daily activities make ample demands on him in the form of physical and manual work, a contrasting hobby is preferable. Depending on your own tastes and fields of interest, collecting of any kind affords an absorbing hobby—whether you decide to collect stamps or gramophone records, books or coins, old china or bottle tops. Or you may want to draw or paint. This hobby is attracting more adherents than ever before.

If your day's work has tired your body but not made a heavy tax on your mind, you might try learning a foreign language through records, or outline a course of reading on a subject of major interest to yourself. If you are interested in politics, find out what men are actually representing your interests in local affairs as well as the names of the more important members of the government. Make it a point to follow week by week how they vote, what kind of job they are doing. After a few weeks of digging down for the real facts, you will begin to find this of fascinating interest, the kind of interest that broadens out in all directions. You will want to know more about your community, more about your country, more about international affairs.

CHAPTER SEVENTEEN

How to Live on 24 Hours a Day

THE chapter heading above is the key to this book. Every-one has the same allotment—twenty-four hours. By a little planning and forethought, you can learn how to get the most out of that twenty-four hours; the most in energy, in accomplishment, in pleasure, without rush or exhaustion or anxiety or the confusion that comes with trying to do too much in too little time. The reward of managing time is that you have more time.

The next point about that heading is the words, "to live". Few people live with zest or genuine enjoyment. They are regretting the errors of yesterday, or worrying about the problems of to-morrow, or dreaming of a world in which everything is wonderful, and so escaping altogether from to-day. Or they are tired and nervous and under par so that they are incapable of getting any enjoyment out of the present moment. They are just dragging along. But the only moment you have to live is this one. Not the past, not the future. *Now.*

If you want to achieve this full, zestful living, making use of your energy and getting real pleasure out of the day, there are some simple, common-sense rules for living that will help you to accomplish it.

Set the Clock Ahead

Set your alarm clock ahead ten minutes.

"I am dead tired in the morning," you groan. "Every minute of sleep is precious. Those early morning hours are the ones when I sleep the best."

I know how you feel, but this ten-minute leeway is going to be a big help in starting the day well. Once you get used to it you will never willingly give it up.

How are you to use those ten minutes? By stretching, which will do you more good than the extra sleep. Stretching will help you to overcome the unhealthy morning habits that are at the root of so much tension.

Lie on your back and inhale deeply while you raise your arms, not merely lifting them but stretching them so that you feel the pull in your sides under your arms and down your back. Exhale while you drop them.

After stretching a few times, turn over on your right side and put your right hand on your right shoulder. (See the diagram on page 60.)

Raise the bent arm towards your head while you inhale. You will feel the stretch all the way down to your waist, through your side and back muscles, so that the ribs on your right side seem to have expanded. This is a sign that this part of your lung, which was dormant and lazy, is beginning to participate more fully in your breathing. Repeat the stretch several times and then turn on the other side and give your left side this benefit. Your heart will be grateful for the flexibility which your ribs acquire.

After a few minutes of stretching the upper part of your body, lie on your back, inhale, and stretch your legs, starting at your heel tendons so that your toes move upward. You should feel the stretch from the heels to the small of the back and I promise that this daily repeated stretch will strengthen the lower back muscles in a way that will compensate for the damaging effect of so many hours of sitting. It will also help you to eliminate any lower back aches not caused by internal conditions.

Now it is time to get out of bed. Wait a minute. Take it easy, please!

Don't rush. Don't scramble quickly out of bed. That is like trying to start a car in high gear, throwing a strain on your heart and muscles.

Now try it again. Take your time, and inhale as you start to swing up. You see, that was no effort at all. Keep this in mind whenever you get up from a chair during the day. Try it first by putting a chair in front of a mirror. Watch yourself when you pull up out of a chair in the old way. Now inhale and see how much your appearance is improved as you swing yourself up. The initiative for this movement comes from the knees.

Remember that you have given yourself a few minutes of extra time. Don't rush. You are going to live this day, not tear through it as though it were a steeplechase. Take time for your bath and for healthy toilet habits. Allowing time for evacuation either before or after breakfast is essential for your

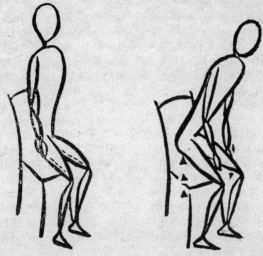

Right   *Wrong*
In rising from a chair, the movement should begin at the knees

health. The person who rushes through his bathroom processes, tense and hurried, blocks proper elimination and suffers for it all the rest of the day.

A Sane Breakfast

What you eat for breakfast is less important than how you

eat it. If you grab a cup of coffee on the run you are throwing your digestive apparatus out of gear and creating tension before the day has even started. Your energy comes from the food you eat. Make it a rule, if it is humanly possible to do so, to sit down for your breakfast and to eat it without haste. Food that you enjoy and eat without hurry will do you more good than the food that you bolt.

Breakfast should be your favourite meal, however much or little you eat. It sets the tempo for the day and creates the frame of mind in which you face your work or your problems.

The principles of relaxation will do you no good if you simply read them and save them, like that book you mean to read when you get around to it, for a leisure hour. They should be applied through every moment of the twenty-four hours and the time to start is at the beginning of the day.

Be on Time

Punctuality, if you make it a rule, will help you to avoid tension. When you are always rushing to catch up with your schedule, you are in a constant state of tension. Start your day rightly by allowing that extra ten minutes. That amount of leeway, slight as it is, gives you a sensation of having extra time for the whole day.

Punctuality has been called the politeness of kings. Since we are a democratic people, let us be polite to ourselves. Punctuality is truly the greatest politeness you can have for yourself, your family, and your friends. The knowledge that you are punctual gives everyone associated with you a feeling of security, of being able to rely on your keeping your appointments.

Children should be taught punctuality from the very beginning. In the first place, the sooner these habits are learned, the easier they are to learn. Second, it will prove of great value to the child himself. This rule should be a strict one. The child must return home at the time he was told to come, or telephone and explain the delay. Carelessness in holding the child to some sense of punctuality will result in the failure of the whole lesson.

Do not make excuses for yourself if you are in the habit of being late. Ask yourself why you fail to be punctual. Did you decide to stay in bed a few minutes longer? Did you go on reading too long because you just wanted to finish the chapter? Was the radio so interesting you could not leave it?

But what happened when you suddenly looked at your watch and discovered that you were going to be late? At that glance at your watch, all your muscles tightened with shock. You dressed hastily, carelessly, spilling things, forgetting things, and dashed out of the house not looking your best and knowing it—a fact that always leaves a person at a disadvantage. You had to pay a heavy penalty in tension, dissatisfaction with yourself, and exhaustion from hurry and the scramble to make your appointment, and all for a few minutes that you could quite easily have allowed yourself.

Plan Your Time

It is an axiom that if you want anything done, ask a busy person to do it. Why? Because the busy person is the one who has time. If you plan your time, you will have more time.

If you rush around complaining that you "never have a minute", you'd better look into the matter. Because you have twenty-four hours a day and that is all the time there is. What are you doing with it?

"Why," you begin indignantly, "I've done this and that, and thus and so. I haven't a minute."

Well, look back and take it hour by hour. If you are quite honest with yourself, you will discover either that there is a surprising amount of time for which you can't account or that the things you were doing in such a rush actually require longer than they should.

What is the trouble? The trouble is planning. Perhaps you have learned how to budget your money, but you haven't learned how to budget the hours and the minutes, the most valuable and irreplaceable gift you have. Not one of those hours or minutes will ever come back. You have to live them and enjoy them as they pass or not at all. You can't do it to-morrow. You can't do it yesterday.

So plan your time to-day. I don't mean that you should allot every minute of it to some particular task, but that you should estimate the amount of time your basic tasks require and then live within that budget. The big executive arranges things so that he has enough leeway for emergencies. He "has time". The little fellow often likes to feel that he is rushed to death, that there isn't a spare moment on his appointment book. He is the one who never catches up and who keeps you waiting indefinitely for an appointment.

Have the courage to see yourself critically and honestly in this respect. Learn to differentiate between the matters that are important and those that are unimportant, and arrange your time accordingly. Don't let the details of living swamp life itself. If you really put your mind on this, you will discover that your appointment book has a few empty spaces, moments in which you can relax, and think at ease about the problems at hand so that you can dispose of them instead of having them clutter your desk, your mind, and your nervous system.

Being rushed is not a virtue in itself. It is merely a sign of bad management. The art of living consists not in stuffing the day as full as possible, but in getting through that day with a sense of achievement, of enjoyment, and without excessive fatigue.

Untidiness Can Cause Tension

Planning, you see, not only helps you to avoid tension and to provide you with more leisure time, but it arranges your twenty-four hours in a more orderly fashion. An orderly plan has an additional value, because it means an orderly mind.

An orderly mind, in turn, is one that functions efficiently

226

and without the mental confusion that leads to a scattering of effort, anxiety, and the tendency to be "all mixed up".

To be orderly is simply to achieve a form of mental discipline. And the first and simplest application of orderliness, the one on which you are judged far more than you ever realise, is the obvious matter of tidiness.

Yes, untidiness is a cause of tension, of cluttered days, of bogging down your twenty-four hours in helpless confusion.

A tidy person goes to bed at night, with his clothes prepared for the next day so that he could even find them in the dark in case of an emergency, such as a fire.

His books and letters, or any object that he wants to take to his office, are kept in a certain spot. All he has to do is to pick them up as he leaves the house. There is no overlooking or forgetting them or wondering where on earth they are, with a resulting frantic scramble at the last moment.

No one, you think confidently, can guess whether or not you are a tidy person. But look around and see how obvious it is in the other fellow; the one who dashed off in the wrong clothes because he hadn't prepared anything for rainy weather; the one who settled down at his desk and realised he left his important papers at home. You can even observe untidiness in a person's movements and walk, because lack of organisation affects both mind and body.

Let's take a look at the behaviour of the untidy person. He drops into bed at night, knowing subconsciously that nothing is prepared for morning.

Next morning, the weather has changed, and he tries to find warmer clothes in a hurry. He remembers that the suit he needs is at the cleaner's, and he should have picked it up a week ago but it slipped his mind.

As he starts to leave the house, he recalls an important document he must take with him. He looks around casually and then in desperation, pawing frantically through the drawers of his desk. He had intended to put it on his desk but he must have dropped it somewhere else.

By now the room looks like a battlefield and the time has

227

passed for breakfast. He closes the jumbled-up drawers and rushes out, without breakfast, reaching his office limp and exhausted. All day he dreads going home because he knows the drawers of his desk are a mess and he will have to straighten them out. And heaven knows how much unfinished business he will find in them!

Not only his mind is confused but his body has been mistreated, because the rapid search made him tense, and his bewildered hunting established wrong switchboard connections from brain to muscles.

Try, from now on, to organise your life and your belongings. The length of time it will take is slight compared with the time consumed in making up for your untidiness; and the calmness and confidence that you derive from this organisation are infinitely worth-while.

Just as children should be taught punctuality, from the beginning, so they should be trained in tidiness. However they may baulk at such discipline now, they will be rewarded for it in later years. Untidiness is one cause of a sense of insecurity. Therefore, be strict with children in this regard and teach them by experience.

The child who repeatedly leaves his toys out of doors in the rain must be taught that he has to go out and get them, even if it entails getting wet, or that the toys will be taken away and not replaced. A few such lessons will be far more effective than constant scolding by a mother who ends by bringing in the toys herself.

System Does It

Just as you budget your money, plan your twenty-four hours. If you do your best thinking at night, plan the day's activities before you go to bed; if you think better in the early morning, do your planning before you get out of bed. Don't simply list in your mind, helter-skelter, all the things that should be done and then look at them in despair, thinking, "I can never in the world manage all that."

Start by looking carefully at the tasks ahead, and separating those which are essential from those which are not essential. Plan for the essential ones, and make up your mind, "I will fit the others in when and if it is convenient, but I won't try to fill every minute. I will allow myself some leeway for emergencies, some moments in which to rest."

Above all, in planning your day, remember that this day can only be lived once, it will never come again. Therefore, you must plan for something during that day that will give you pleasure, something to which you will look forward. This may be a luncheon engagement with a friend, a book you have set aside for the evening, a radio feature you want to hear. Whether it is small or large, every day should have some pleasure. To defraud yourself of that enjoyment because you are "too busy" is to miss the whole point of living.

You will find it a big help to put your day's schedule in writing, or at least to make a written list of the things you must accomplish. Paper and pencil kept at the bedside are most convenient if you do your planning the first thing in the morning. Check off each item as you do it. You will discover that there is a wonderful feeling about crossing off that list and destroying the paper, knowing that everything has been done.

As we have pointed out, the unaccomplished task causes a residual tension. Therefore, it is wise to plan to do the unpleasant things as soon as you can and get them out of the way: a visit to the dentist, a bill you have put off paying, the cupboard you dislike cleaning. When they are done, you will experience a sensation of relief, and also the feeling of strength that comes with having tackled the unpleasant job. Each such victory leaves you with a greater sense of strength and with more self-reliance.

The Work-day

Relaxation is where you find it. Throughout this book I have pointed out how you get tired and how you can learn

229

to overcome your fatigue and prevent it. The ideal system, I said, was to check it as you go along.

For a few weeks, until your new habits become automatic, watch yourself at work. Be aware of the way you sit and stand and walk; be conscious of the reason for your aches and pains. Ask yourself what made you tired. What were you doing wrong? What muscle groups were over-worked and which ones were under-worked?

Relax *as you go along*. In time, you should be able to work in a state of relaxation. Meantime, watch to see whether you are growing tense and, if so, let go. This is not a time-consumer, it is a time-saver. It means that you will end your work-day rested instead of being fatigued and depressed.

If it is possible to get a few minutes of complete rest, both morning and afternoon, fine! If not, when you go to the cloakroom, make use of the time to yawn and stretch, to pull yourself up against the wall for a sense of proper alignment.

Before you go out to lunch, take a few minutes for a couple of long breaths and feel yourself let go from head to foot. If it is possible, eat without rush in a quiet place.

If you ride to and from work, however noisy or crowded your surroundings, close your eyes to rest them and allow yourself those minutes or that hour—whatever it may be—for silence and meditation.

Silence Saves Your Strength

All of us need intervals in which we do no talking. To be silent for a short interval during the day is an important source of strength-saving. Talking requires far more breath and energy than most people realise. It is a strenuous occupation, even—perhaps especially—if it is the uncontrolled chatter commonly ascribed to women, but as frequently found in men.

Watch yourself for a few days and find out how large a share you take in the conversation. Perhaps you are one of those extreme cases, a person who has to be a monologist and carry the conversation single-handed, a quality that always leads to tension. How much that you had to say was important or interesting to anyone but yourself? Watch others and you will see that the people who are most successful and who accomplish the most are those who know how to be silent. They focus their shot, they don't scatter it.

Naturally, I do not suggest that you become a Trappist monk. Simply realise that unnecessary conversation is a waste of energy, a drain on your nerves, and creates tension. When you are completely relaxed, you are willing to be silent and to enjoy it.

There is one daily and constant source of tension that leads to exhaustion, yet is rarely suspected. That is the abuse of the telephone. People who spend hours chattering over the telephone are seldom conscious of the strain it causes them. One reason is the physical strain of keeping the phone pressed against the ear with one hand. Another reason is the mental strain, of which nearly everyone is unconscious, of attempting to guess, from the voice alone, all the changes of mood of the person to whom you are talking, without the help of seeing his changing expression or gestures. It is a kind of jigsaw puzzle, in which the listener tries to piece together a picture without sufficient clues.

On your return home, you should allow a few minutes of complete rest before you eat your evening meal. Lie down if you can, let yourself go, and breathe deeply. Before you get up, stretch as you did in the morning. You will feel refreshed and ready for a pleasant evening.

If you adopt this sort of routine, based on a planned day in which you do not try to do more than you can handle, you will find that you will have little trouble with insomnia when you go to bed.

Chief Subject of Conversation

The purpose of the foregoing rules of living is to point

the way to spend twenty-four hours every day and enjoy it. It should be normal for you to feel well, to feel buoyantly cheerful, without aches and pains.

Life is not an indeterminate sentence, it is an adventure. People in general are so far below their own health potentialities that they take lack of energy and vitality and zest as their normal condition. That simply isn't so. With few exceptions, you can make yourself feel infinitely better than you do.

Pay attention for a few days to the talk you hear around you, at home, at work, at parties, on the street. You will discover that the chief subject of conversation is illness, insomnia, aches and pains, operations, all the endless variety of health problems. Some people would actually prefer to talk about it than to do something about it. On the whole, it is good advice to make it a rule not to talk about your health. The temptation to cap the story of your friend who slept only four hours last night with your own experiences of a harrowing night in which you never closed your eyes will be almost irresistible. But don't give in to it.

If there is really something wrong with your health, something beyond the wrong functioning that comes with your faulty habits, don't speculate about it, or take the advice of your friends, or prescribe your own remedies, or worry for fear it is this or that.

See Your Doctor

Some people have lived below par for so long that they take poor health for granted. They do not realise that with the enormous progress in our knowledge of nutrition and vitamins, which shows how to overcome so many pains and fatigues due to deficiencies, the doctor can help them to restore themselves to good health. That is what the doctor is for. It is what he is trained to do and eager to do. And yet the doctor is still forced to say too often, "If only you had come to see me sooner!"

If your doctor discovers that you have a chronic ailment which he can help but not cure, take time to think your situation through clearly. If you feel worried and uncertain, get a second medical opinion. But when you know that you have a gall-bladder or kidney condition or a stomach ulcer, do your talking to your doctor, and not to your friends. Find out how you should adjust your life, what kind of diet and regime you are expected to follow. Discuss this with your family so they will understand what is necessary and then tell yourself, "I am lucky to have found a doctor who got to the root of my troubles. I know what I must do and that I am getting the right treatment. Now, I'll devote the rest of my time and energy to living and not spend it talking to other people about my symptoms."

Easy? I didn't say it was easy. But let me tell you the story of a friend of mine who, for nearly thirty years, was rarely free from pain, because she suffered from a glandular condition about which doctors knew nothing until very recently. Her suffering was so acute that she had to have morphine to relieve her pain and often fainted during these attacks. And yet she gave the world the impression of health and energy. Having seen her in one of these attacks, I asked, "How is it possible for you to be so cheerful and to give others so much courage?"

She smiled. "When I was very young," she said, "I was expecting a baby and several medical authorities told my husband that there was no hope of saving either my life or my child's. By a miracle I pulled through and my child is now grown up and a fine person. Knowing how near death I had been, I made a vow that, whatever happened to me, I would always be thankful that I had been allowed to live. And I have tried to keep my vow. That is why I was able to take even my pain without letting it get me down mentally. I reminded myself that at least I was alive. And now the doctors have learned to understand the condition and to relieve my suffering."

She pondered for a moment and laughed. "What a waste

233

of mental energy it would have been if I had let those thirty years of pain make me sorry for myself!''

You will get out of your twenty-four hours pretty much what you put into them. It depends on you whether they will be rewarding or a burden.

CHAPTER EIGHTEEN

Hints to Housewives

WHAT should the housewife know about her daily routine that will keep her relaxed and healthy? If you are a housewife, you have an immense advantage over the desk worker—whether typist or top-management executive—in that your daily activities call for variety and for the kind of bending and stretching movements that help to keep your muscles flexible. Your fatigue and nerve tension, as a rule, have other sources than those of the sedentary worker. While there are many exceptions, in general the reasons are:

1. Wrong physical habits of work
2. Wrong organisation of work
3. The dullness of routine
4. A feeling that you do not receive enough appreciation

Planning the Day

The housewife has another advantage over the employee. That is, she is her own boss and she can plan her day with a view to her own convenience and in the way she wants to do it.

The essential thing is that you should have a plan and follow it. Here, too, you must learn how to distinguish between the essential and the unessential job. If you find yourself worn out at the end of the day, try to figure out exactly how you used your energy.

Did you plan too much, so that you were rushing all day long, trying to keep up with an impossible schedule? If so, what did you try to do that could have been left for another day?

Did you work inefficiently, bustling back and forth from room to room, upstairs and down, picking up one object at a time and taking it to its proper place? An immense amount of fatigue in housework comes from a total lack of efficiency. From puttering.

In planning your day, there are major time elements to mark off. That is, you know in advance the time at which meals should be served. You know what you intend to serve. Therefore, you can estimate the approximate amount of time that must be spent in shopping and in preparing the meals. By roughing out your menus for a week in advance and doing your shopping for staples once or twice a week, you can cut down greatly on the time spent in shopping, particularly that anxious last-minute buying when you scan the shelves in the grocer's wondering frantically, "Oh, *what* shall I get for dinner?"

The knowledge that you have planned nothing, that you are leaving it to the last minute, and that, however long you put it off, you must inevitably serve some kind of meal, will keep you tense all day long. Taking a half-hour once a week to do your planning will put you at ease and give you more serenity.

Your housework needs the same kind of organisation as your menus. Think it out in advance and let planning save you a lot of needless running back and forth.

Varying the Jobs

Whether you have a whole house or a small apartment, there is variety in your jobs, from cooking to making beds, from dusting to pressing your clothes, from rearranging the furniture to gardening.

All these tasks sum up not to thankless drudgery but to making a home. You are your own boss. Plan your day so that there will be variety. If you have to do a lot of bending and stretching while you clean or wash, let the next job be darning and mending or going over the household accounts, a job at which you can sit down. Don't approach your housework as though it were a punishment meted out by an unkind fate. Make it fun by doing it the way you *like* doing it. If there is a favourite radio programme at the time when you usually do your morning dishes, leave them until after lunch and do your darning while you hear the programme you enjoy. Remember that you are planning your day not only for more efficiency and more relaxation, but so that you can enjoy living it.

A housewife who plans her work properly is in the same fortunate position as the farmer, whose work also requires a constant change in body movement and a maximum of independence. Housework should be planned to bring a constant and healthy change from standing to sitting.

Instead of dreading the exertion of bed-making and hanging clothes, you will be wise to understand that these very activities help to keep you in good health and good spirits. Curiously enough, the women who complain most about these jobs are frequently the ones who will pay high prices for exercise courses in reducing which, basically, simply give them the same sort of muscular work-out.

Right Habits

If you have tried lifting and stretching in the proper way, as described in previous chapters, you have learned to enjoy the freedom and ease which these movements give you, and you understand why I say that the housewife lives a far healthier life than the women who are forced to sit for eight hours doing sedentary work, or standing all day behind a counter. Instead of taxing your muscles and tiring you, the right kind of lifting and stretching while you do your housework actually helps to relax and rest you, to keep you limber and your body younger.

For the next few weeks, watch your habits of doing things and be careful to substitute right for wrong habits in all bodily movements. You will be aware of increased comfort from the beginning, and if you are strict with yourself the right movements will become a habit sooner than you expect.

How to Work

For instance, when you are hanging up clothes or making beds, remember to inhale as you lift your arms. The movement will flow as though your arms were flying, and there will be less tax on your system. The right muscles will come into use with less strain on your heart and your whole system will be grateful for the increased flexibility, which, in turn, will affect your spirits and improve your mood.

When you lift a basket of laundry, protect your back from injury by inhaling first, and hold your breath while you are carrying the basket. If you have to go too far, set down the basket while you exhale and lift it again on the next inhaling. The moment's time required to set it down is more than compensated for by the amount of strength you save in this way.

In reaching up to a high shelf or screwing in electric light bulbs, inhale as you raise your arm and you will avoid the usual unpleasant feeling of strain and pulling.

This breathing routine throughout your working day will keep you physically young and flexible beyond your years, and help to keep you young and fresh in mind. It will also prevent the many aches and pains women are apt to get in middle age for no other reason than the stiffness and inflexibility that come of doing their daily routine activities in the wrong way.

Mopping floors, sweeping, vacuuming and carpet sweeping should all be done with a swinging rhythm, based on inhaling and exhaling. Make this a real rhythm, so that your body really sways with the motion. No, don't say that it is a bother to think of how you do your work. As a matter of fact, once you bring yourself to the point of changing your habits—and it is that mental decision which is hard; people hate to change their habits—you will find that all the physical processes are

238

much easier for you. Not only that, but they make you feel fresher, more vigorous, more alive. That's a wonderful feeling.

How often my pupils have exclaimed in chagrin, "Why weren't we taught from childhood the right way to do things so that we could enjoy them? We've been tiring ourselves out for nothing." Unless you are a professional martyr, and there are a lot of them, you will find that you can give your life more savour and zest by improving your physical habits. A body that functions at its peak means not only an efficient person but a happy one. Try it and see!

Carrying Children

Many young mothers strain themselves or get over-tired by carrying heavy babies or small children. Never lift the child without inhaling first.

And here's a trick that is a great help. If the baby is old enough to hold on around your neck, and you have to carry him for any distance, carry him on your back. You will find this far easier and less strenuous than trying to hold a heavy child in your arms.

Both the Indians and the Orientals have always carried their children in this way. And I have seen many young parents in Europe start out on hiking trips, carrying a child on their backs in a sort of knapsack, a piece of sturdy canvas with holes for the child's legs. It works, too. Try to carry a heavy child on your back and you will be astonished to see how much less tiring this method is.

Rest Periods

When you have planned your day so that you are not attempting to do too much, and you have eliminated all the time wasted in puttering and inefficiency, you will discover that you have free periods. Your first use of these must be for rest. Remember that fatigue must be forestalled and prevented *as you go along*.

Take five minutes in the middle of the morning. That's not much, is it? Not as much time as you spent looking at the ads in the morning paper or listening to a radio programme or gossiping over the telephone. Lie down and let yourself go. Let your jaw drop and your eyes "fall back" in your head. Listen to your slow, deep breathing and feel the air wash through you like a great wave.

Before you dress to do your marketing in the afternoon, give yourself another five minutes of complete rest. This is not a waste of time; it is a saving, in the long run, both of time and of energy. It is a clever way of keeping yourself in the best possible shape so that you will be able to enjoy the next step in your work. Try it and you will be astonished to find what these five-minute rest periods in your daily routine can do for you.

If you are the lucky owner of a back porch or a garden, lie down out of doors. Don't look around your garden or your bedroom and worry about the things that should be done— the lawn that needs mowing or the mirror that should be polished—that's not the idea. Keep your eyes closed and try to empty your mind of thoughts. Your work has been planned so you have neither mental confusion nor worry about that. This time is yours in which to regain and affirm your own inward serenity and peace.

Help for Your Hands

The average housewife has her hands in hot water many times a day and as a rule she follows this immersion by rubbing her hands with some lotion to keep them lubricated and soft.

When doing this to your hands, take a couple of minutes to examine your finger joints. The first joint, below the fingernail, is especially exposed to damage as a result of having the hands in hot water—washing dishes several times a day, doing laundry, cooking and cleaning.

Is this first joint shiny? When you touch the skin, does it

240

have a leatherish texture? Is the joint easy to move and flexible so that you can bend it at a right angle?

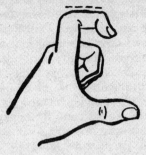

How to bend the finger to make its joints more flexible

The tightness of the tissue over this joint is often the cause not only of what you think is arthritis in your hands, but of arm and shoulder pains as well. You can help yourself to improve the condition of these joints in three different ways:

1. With thumb and forefinger start an easy, rotating movement just below the nails on the opposite hand, massaging the joint on top, bottom, and both sides.

2. Move the joint up and down and try to bend it at a right angle. The skin will redden and, after a time, the joint will feel loose. That is what we are working to achieve.

3. Now shake your wrists up and down rapidly several times, letting the fingers hang loose. Try to make a practice of doing this each time you have finished with the dishes and the laundry.

Housework Is So Dull

What can you do to avoid the boredom of doing routine work over and over again?

Boredom, as we pointed out in an earlier chapter, is a reflection of your own attitude. Almost every activity or profession, however glamorous its outward appearance, has its long periods of repetitive routine. Consider for a moment the life of an actor or actress—one of the more glamorous professions. If you have ever sat in a bleak unheated and empty theatre listening to a cast rehearsing a play, hour after hour, day in and day out, you will realise that behind the footlights and the applause there are hours of the dullest of routine. The actor who was bored by it would be poor in actual performance. His thoughts are on perfecting his work with a view to a fine performance.

In the same way, the housewife who straightens her living-room with a sense of acute boredom is setting the stage for a dull home. If she had in mind the appearance of the tidy room, and considered ways and means of making it more attractive, more pleasant for her family—setting the stage, as it were, for the evening performance when her family is gathered around her—she would not be bored. For, make no mistake about it, a clever woman sets the emotional tone of her family. If her husband and children return to find her bored, tired, restless and dissatisfied, full of complaints, the amount of housework she has done will be of little avail in creating a home atmosphere. Her children will make every effort to get out of the house for the evening, and the relations between husband and wife will be of an unpleasant nature.

You can relieve the sense of routine by varying your work schedule from day to day so that every day has some individual task or pleasure in it and you don't have that sense of "the same old thing". Hours of ironing are lightened by having a radio at hand.

It is often possible to find a solution to the boredom of housework by getting together with your neighbours who have the same, or similar, problems. You may be able to work out some sort of co-operative system by which you will take turns baby-sitting for the group, thus allowing the others an afternoon or evening of leisure and freedom.

Help for the Young Housewife

One of the problems that have developed as a result of

women's emancipation is the difficulty many young house-wives find, after going to college or working for a couple of years, in adjusting themselves to being tied down to the care of their babies. On the job and at college, they had week-ends or free days to spend as they pleased. But the housewife has a seven-day week. While she loves her husband, wants her children and her home, she chafes at her lack of freedom, at having no time for herself, at the impossibility of change.

In some cases, an understanding mother or mother-in-law will be able to ease this tension by taking over the children once in a while; or a neighbourhood group may take turns at handling the problem for a number of young mothers.

Instead of building up resentment and therefore tension over this problem—which affects millions of young mothers—talk it over with your husband, your family, and your neigh-bours. Among them some remedy should be worked out that will give you your free time each week.

The Pitch Pipe

In the days of our grandparents, the leader of a choral group or a choir had a pitch pipe which set the tone for the group. In the family, it is the mother who, like a pitch pipe, sets the tone for her small group, a tone that may be loud and discordant, or harmonious and restful. In a way, she sets that tone literally by the pitch of her own voice. If it is high, querulous and whining, or loud and angry, the result is tension for her family. If her voice is modulated and con-trolled, she helps to prevent tension.

But for the most part, she sets the tone of her home and the mood of her family by her own mood. That mood is a reflection of her mental and emotional state, which in turn frequently reflect her physical condition. If she is worn out, nervous and tense, these qualities will appear in her attitude toward her family. There is little happiness or comfort or peace or rest in coming home to a wife and mother who greets you with the groan, "I am simply worn out".

While there are always trying days in anyone's life, the routine of running a house can be managed without exhausting the housewife. And yet I can imagine the anger, the tears and the resentment of the woman who, when she complained, was told, "Then why don't you learn how to manage better?"

Over and over again I have repeated—because it is of such tremendous importance—that the person who is in his best health is also in his best spirits. The quest for happiness, like the quest for the blue bird in Maeterlinck's play, ends at home.

According to our dreams and the fairy tales, whose aura too many adults carry about with them, happiness comes through the wave of a wand by a fairy godmother; good fortune falls into our laps; Cinderella wins her prince; the poor boy, like a Horatio Alger hero, marries the boss's daughter and is rich ever after. And the books and the films too often end with wedding bells and the assumption of the fairy story, "And so they lived happily ever after".

But the wedding bells are not the end of the adventure. They are the beginning. Happiness, in an adult world, does not come with the spilling on to the carpet of a gleaming money bag, or of a chemist's preparation that will make you beautiful, or a gland extract that will keep you perennially young. Adult happiness means health, peace of mind, the full expression of yourself in a rounded personality, and the wonderful ability to enjoy being alive. It means mutual giving and receiving.

Lack of Appreciation

And here, I think, the housewife has her most legitimate complaint. The employee who does a good job gets a rise or a better position or, at the least, a word of praise from the boss. But too often the housewife suffers from a lack of appreciation. The family takes for granted that the house will be clean and the beds made and the meals cooked.

There is nothing more depressing than lack of recognition. According to expert analysts of labour troubles, the first requirement of the worker is not salary but recognition of himself as an individual and of his work as being useful. What, then, about the housewife?

Surely it is a small thing for the family to recognise the need and the right of the housewife for appreciation of her efforts. Praise for a good meal, thanks for freshly laundered shirts, a compliment on the appearance of a room—little things, aren't they, and so easily done. Yet how often does it occur to the husband or the children to notice these things and to express their pleasure and appreciation for them? Children are taught to say "thank you" as a matter of politeness. Certainly, they should be taught to carry this attitude a little farther, to realise that the attentions and comforts they receive are the result of a woman's thought and effort. I do not mean, naturally, that the situation should be distorted so that the mother demands praise and thanks for every gesture she makes. But there is a happy medium which should make almost every home a more harmonious place than it is.

If the woman is to draw on her own energy and her own courage to keep her home a cheerful place and a place of peace, let her know, at least, what that peace means to you —and occasionally, tell her that you are grateful.

CHAPTER NINETEEN

How to Get More Out of Life

WHILE each of us regards himself as a unique being, unlike anyone else, we are, taking it by and large, very much alike. We are all seeking the same basic things out of life:

> Health
> Security
> Love
> Self-expression
> Peace of mind

And these things sum up to the state of mind which we call happiness.

Our Neurotic World

Lewis Browne opened his book, *This Believing World*, with the telling phrase: "In the beginning there was fear." He was referring to the very dawn of civilisation and the frightened struggles of primitive man against his environment, against the hostile forces of nature, of wild animals, and savage men. But to-day, after the passage of unmeasured thousands of years, after the slow and painful growth of a high form of civilisation, man is still afraid. As acutely afraid as he has ever been. And he is sick with his fear. But we know at last that the fear complex under which we live is not in the world but in ourselves. Until the individual can learn to live in harmony with himself, without tension, he cannot create harmony in his immediate surroundings, with his family or his co-workers; and certainly he cannot create international peace. For peace starts with the individual. It starts with *you*.

When the Blows Fall

It is apparent to any adult mind that the peace so deeply longed for by all of us comes not simply by an escape from the situations which threaten or disturb that peace—whether into narcotics or dreams or within oneself. It comes from the fortitude and self-reliance that can create peace in a troubled world. No human being can be so fortunate as to live a life without trouble. His triumph comes in learning how to take it. Let me hasten to add that I do not mean by that to make himself a long-suffering martyr. Far from it. What we are aiming at is not martyrdom but triumphant happiness.

And so we come back to our main subject of relaxation. Why? Because when we achieve real relaxation we achieve flexibility, not only of our body but of our mind. And mental flexibility is the only real strength when the blows fall.

Every day we see disaster strike at people whom we regarded as secure, invulnerable. The death of a beloved person, the loss of health or money or home and country. Some of these people crack up and some of them seem to acquire new strength and courage. Why?

The curious thing is that it is often the so-called strong man who succumbs to the blow; it is the quiet, inconspicuous person who weathers the storm. Again, why?

Well, observe the trees in your garden or in a park when a great storm strikes them. From the window you see your big, strong trees standing proudly against the onslaught of the wind, while your willows bow before it, bending so far that you fear they will never be able to straighten up again. But when the wind has died down and the sun comes out, you go to view the damage. You find that your strong proud trees have snapped off because they could not bend and therefore reduce the power of the wind. But the willows have

247

sprung back into position because they were flexible enough to take the blow.

So, with people, there is a difference in the way the blow is received. Say that a serious illness develops. The tense person has fewer resources for recuperation than the flexible one.

True Relaxation

Relaxation, therefore, means far more than supple muscles and freedom from fatigue. It means the ability to bend with the storm, to adjust yourself to unforeseen difficulties. It is your safest insurance in the face of the eventualities fate may bring into your life. For with this flexibility comes self-reliance; a freedom from the fear of the future which spoils to-day for so many people. The tense person wonders, "What will happen to me?" The flexible person thinks confidently, "Whatever it is, I can take it". He has acquired a courage of the spirit.

Some years ago a middle-aged woman came to me, suffering with liver trouble and such fatigue that she was exhausted after a few steps. She had recently lost her husband and after a lifetime of protection and freedom from responsibility, she had been thrown on her own resources. As a result, her worry and distrust of herself and the future had made her ill. She was old beyond her years and shrank at the responsibility that had been thrust upon her.

As we began to relieve her tension—by the very same methods explained in this book—she gained in self-confidence. Some seven years after our work together, I met her in the street. She was buoyant and happy and looked younger than when I had first seen her. She told me that she had re-married, but not a marriage which would make life easier for her or relieve her of responsibility. She had married a widower with six children and she was looking after his big house in the country.

"I am so grateful," she said, "that I learned how to relax and get the most out of my energy. Otherwise, I would never

248

have had the courage to take on so much responsibility and I would have lost all this happiness." For the marriage had turned out to be a real success, not only for her, but for her husband and stepchildren too.

How Are You Doing?

After you have been applying the techniques in this book for a short period—say, three weeks—ask yourself the following questions, which will serve as a check on your improved ability to relax and its effect on your ability to live:

1. Can you take a joke on yourself and laugh whole-heartedly?
2. Can you forget a hurt or do you bear a grudge?
3. Do you first see the good in a person or is your primary reaction critical?
4. Are you afraid of competition?
5. Are you suspicious?
6. Can you listen with interest and concentration to others or are you quickly bored unless you can talk about yourself?
7. Are you afraid to make decisions?
8. Are you able to take the consequences of your own actions without blaming the outcome on others?
9. Are you content to be yourself or would you rather be someone else?

Living With Others

Not long ago, a New York newspaper carried the caption:

"IN-LAW DISEASE HITS BRITAIN: HOUSING ITS ONLY CURE."

According to the story, an English hospital had reported that one out of every hundred patients was suffering from illnesses whose basis was conflicts arising from having to share a house with a mother-in-law. The symptoms varied from hysterics to exhaustion, but the cause was the same.

Of all the hazards of living, the greatest is undoubtedly the people with whom we have to live. Obviously, we cannot

249

make them over. The only thing we can do about the situation is to become so relaxed that the impact of others will not arouse tensions in us, to be so flexible that, like the willow, we can bend before the irritation and straighten up after it has passed.

One of my pupils was a woman of early middle-age who had a husband and two small children. She complained of the confinement, of never having any time free from her children.

"But," I suggested, "why can't your husband take them to the park and entertain them on Saturday afternoons, giving you this time to yourself?"

She shook her head. "It wouldn't do. The children make him so nervous that he never plays with them. He is in a constant state of jitters for fear they will hurt themselves if they get a bit rough when they are playing."

At my suggestion, she asked her husband to come to see me and we began to work releasing tension. We had been working at it only three weeks when he came in to see me on a Monday morning. He was beaming.

"Well," he said, "you can't guess how I spent the weekend. I looked after the children while my wife went away. We went out to the park and I've never had so much fun in my life. I didn't worry about them at all, just enjoyed playing with them."

His wife told me later that he had taken to playing with the children when he came home at nights, not only creating a warm relationship with them and happiness for himself, but enabling his wife to have some relief from her long hours with them.

Our Different Rhythms

One way to avoid future tensions and emotional maladjustments is to discover before marriage something about the personal rhythm of your future spouse. For two people of totally different rhythm to attempt to mate is usually as impracticable as to team up a cart horse with a race horse.

Find out whether you enjoy being alone with your partner at a time when you are reading or writing. Do you feel relaxed or does it make you nervous to be with him? Do you enjoy walking together or does one of you want to rush ahead and the other to lag behind?

You may feel that where there is love enough this difference in rhythms does not matter. That may be true, but only if you take that difference into consideration and do not try to ignore it. Learn to adapt yourself so that your two rhythms can function without a lack of harmony.

Let's take an example. Suppose that you are the kind of person who is most alert in the early morning and are ready to get up at six o'clock and get to work. Your partner is a night owl, who is at his best in the afternoon and evening, but likes to sleep late in the morning. If you attempt to adjust your rhythm to his or to force him to adjust his rhythm to yours, there will be dissension and lack of harmony. One of you is being forced to live in a way that is in opposition to his own nature.

Try then to work out an intelligent adjustment. If you want to get up early, do so and go quietly about your affairs, knowing that you are doing what you like doing, and there is no reason for resentment.

These small adjustments are easy to make if you talk them over, understand your differences, and attempt to make a reasonable compromise that will be fair to both. It is little things that cause most of the serious trouble: the fact that one person is tidy and another careless; that one likes to have the radio on and the other is disturbed. These differences lead to tension and quarrels and upset homes when a little good will can work out an adjustment.

The Wrong Politeness

The essential thing in making these adjustments is that you analyse the situation and then talk it out frankly. So much trouble and unhappiness is brought about because of the wrong politeness, keeping these sources of irritation to yourself instead of indicating what they are and trying to find an intelligent and fair solution to them.

Politeness, after all, is only a form of consideration for others. And this brings me to another point, the fact that an ignorance of what constitutes true politeness leads to a sense of insecurity and inferiority. It is essential that children should be trained from the beginning in the rudiments of politeness so that they will feel at ease and not at a disadvantage with other people. I am not talking about the rules of etiquette. The important things are consideration toward others and a sense of security in oneself.

Children should learn not to yell and slam doors when their mother is resting. They should be taught not to leave their rooms untidy in the morning because it is a lack of consideration for their mother, suggesting that the dirty work is good enough for her. They should be brought up to help with the housework and the dishes; they all enjoy their home and their meals, and therefore it should be natural for them to participate in the work these things require.

Most of the tensions in family life grow out of little things, lack of consideration for one another, lack of politeness, careless wounds given in a moment of thoughtless annoyance. It is disheartening to see a quarrelsome and rude family suddenly become polite when guests arrive. There is no place where politeness is so necessary as in the home if it is to be harmonious and self-respecting. The person who is allowed to be rude, careless, thoughtless, and insulting at home and adopts a totally different manner of politeness and consideration outside the home, subconsciously regards this politeness as artificial and dishonest, a disguise covering his real self. In other words, he does not really believe in consideration.

Our False Values

The chances are that you have a desk or dresser drawer which contains a bunch of rusty keys. You have long since moved away from the house whose doors they fitted, or lost the suitcases they locked, or you have forgotten what they were for originally. But you don't throw them away, you have the vague idea "They may come in handy sometime".

Up in the attic or down in the basement or stacked on the shelves of a cupboard you have broken clocks and old magazines, the toys that your son outgrew twenty years ago, and letters from a school friend whose face you have forgotten. You hang on to them though they are of no use to you or to anyone.

In your mind there is stored a lot of rubbish that you have long since outgrown—old wives' tales and superstitions and outmoded ideas and sets of values that have no bearing on the present world. Why don't you look them over in the light of the person you are to-day and discard the ones that are of no further use to you? All that mental clutter prevents clear thinking, just as a jumbled bureau drawer makes it impossible to see at a glance what you have in it and whether it is in condition to wear.

Perhaps the things that change most rapidly are basic values. In the Victorian days, the essential value was "keeping up appearances". With the advent of Horatio Alger, there emerged the "success" value. All that mattered was getting rich, getting to be the head of the firm, having more than your neighbour.

We know to-day that "keeping up appearances" is a shallow business at best, and that money creates neither happiness nor peace of mind. And we have come to realise that the real values that make life rewarding are a healthy body and a peaceful mind. And yet that clutter in the attic of our mind keeps us from seeing clearly. We read in the papers of the fall of great fortunes, and we see the discontent of the wealthy, and the idea that money can create happiness still influences many people.

The New Understanding of Life

Basically, values have changed more rapidly in the last decade than ever before in history. After the fire and dust of the European holocaust had died down and we saw the wreckage, we learned that we must view the years ahead in a different way. The elements we called security are gone; our security has become a matter of our own inner strength. Possessions can vanish over-night. They are not permanent. The accumulation of belongings and luxury no longer seems particularly admirable at a time when hundreds of millions of people must be fed and sheltered.

But along with this knowledge, has come a new awareness of ourselves, a new understanding that there are richer potentialities for happiness within us than we have ever dreamed, opportunities for a more complete flowering of the human personality into its full expression than we ever guessed was possible.

In the main, all the earlier values—the quest for a fortune or for power—were man's groping substitutes to compensate for a lack in himself.

So to-day we are taking a greater interest than ever before in the development of the personality. For the most part, the popular approach has been to surface things: personality was taken to mean your looks and your popularity. But it is infinitely more than that: it is you—body and mind and emotions—living at your peak.

This view of the personality and its infinite and unguessed potentialities is only slowly emerging. Little by little, scientists, experimenting in the field, are coming to the conclusion that only the rare individual has ever tapped his own resources. Man has carried on a constant war with himself in which he is always the loser, mind, body, and emotions carrying on a struggle and out of harmony with each other. And yet there seems sound reason to believe that the fused personality, in which all these elements are in balance and in harmony, has potentialities for self-expression and for happiness beyond our wildest dreams.

The Scientific Production of Love

The chief exponent of this new and exhilarating idea was

Dr. Roger Vittoz, who practised medicine in Switzerland. A detailed account of his experiments appeared in the *Saturday Review of Literature* in 1948, in an article by John F. Wharton, an article which deserves widespread attention because within it lies the seed not only of personal happiness but of international peace as well.

The conclusions reached by Dr. Vittoz were—greatly simplified—as follows:

When the human personality is completely fused—that is, when mind, emotions, and body are working in harmony—the person is not only without fear but is also able to make decisions easily, and frequently taps a source of creative ability of which he was completely unaware.

Dr. Vittoz pointed out that we are conscious of our body when we are ill but not when we are well; that we think about ourselves when we are worried or unhappy and consequently that we are unable to be as kind to others as we would like to be.

But if the personality is really fused and in harmony, we are happy. *We cannot be otherwise.* And just as the healthy person is not concerned with himself, so the happy person is not concerned with his own emotions. He co-operates with others, he gives his love to others, because he cannot help himself.

Relaxation and Peace of Mind

Ministers, educators, and physicians are all trying to find a solution for the problems of tensions, fatigue and fear that have become mass problems. Counselling, psycho-analysis, and psychiatry are being more widely used.

But they tend too often to overlook the fact that a person can only be treated as a whole—body, mind, and emotions. As long as the body remains tense through wrong muscular habits, psycho-analysis will be only partly successful, because the habitual muscular strains will continue to set up new tensions.

One of the first results of applied relaxation through proper muscle use is a clearing of the brain itself: "I can concentrate better than I did; I don't forget things so often; I seem to have more time."

A second, and perhaps more important, result of right body function and physical flexibility, is the effect on the memory and the release of the subconscious. A person who learns how to relax completely—or meditate, as the Eastern teachers call it—acquires the capacity of freeing himself from fears and useless brooding over bad experiences. These experiences do not retreat into his subconscious and do their destructive work, but instead, the person who is physically flexible through complete relaxation can cast them off, be really free. He is able to start a new life again and again, as the willow is able to straighten up after the wind has passed. This wonderful capacity to greet every day and every experience unburdened and unshackled by the past is the real secret of eternal youth.

The whole period of applied relaxation is based on the idea of peaceful living and the capacity for meditation. It is apparent that our Western mode of life makes it impossible for us to adopt the Eastern systems of relaxation without compromise and adaptation to our particular needs. None the less, the methods described in this book make it possible even for people living in crowded cities to achieve the same peace of mind that Eastern religions accomplish under completely different conditions.

Changing Yourself

A real peace movement can come only when people find peace in themselves and learn to establish peace in their family groups. We have the knowledge. We know that science has given us the equipment for the fusion of the personality and the unity of mind and body. We know the benefits of proper nutrition, of psychiatry, and the influence of a relaxed body which uses its breath and its energies to its full capacity.

What we need is the will to extend this knowledge to the next generation, educating them for peaceful living.

We all want peace. We all want security. We all want health and love and happiness. All we need is the will to attain them.

Of all the vices that trouble mankind, perhaps the deadliest is sloth. Laziness. Inertia.

"I know," you say, "it sounds like a good idea. I really am sick of feeling run down. I hate being so tired. I know I am missing a lot by being anxious and fear-ridden. Of course, I want to be happy. But——"

But, you mean, it entails changing a habit. It entails making up your mind to a course of action and then doing something about it. It entails effort.

Within you is the seed of all the things to which you aspire. Give it a chance to grow.